Praise for *Gentling:*
A Practical Guide to Treating PTSD in Abused Children

"William Krill reminds us that 'gentleness is free', but the methodology and philosophy he puts into designing a protocol for treating stress disordered children is priceless. In this book Krill directly addresses identifying stress symptoms, diagnosis and assessment tools, behavioral interpretation and a specific course of treatment to gently guide children from a place of panic, fear and defensiveness to one of a self-empowered transcendence that engages a child's natural impulse to learn. In this world where children are often disenfranchised in trauma care—and all too often treated with the same techniques as adults—Krill makes a compelling case for how to adapt proven post-trauma treatment to the world of a child."

—Michele Rosenthal, HealMyPTSD.com

"William Krill's *Gentling* is one of the most remarkable books I've ever read. The author's approach to treating PTSD in abused children employs a common sense oriented treatment that will not only help the child but will direct the clinician through the 'where do I go next?' question. This book is so needed in the world of PTSD and provides step-by-step understanding and treatment of the battered child. A must read and apply for all counselors, clinicians or anyone who is presented with the painful question, 'What can I do to help this child?'"

—Marjorie McKinnon, Author of
Repair for Kids: A Children's Program for Recovery from Incest and Childhood Sexual Abuse

"Congratulations to Krill when he says that 'being gentle' cannot be over-emphasized in work with the abused. Gentling paired with tolerance on the one hand and clear boundaries on the other will give a victim the space to begin recovery. The former emphasizes non-threatening and the latter promotes safety."

Andrew D. Gibson, PhD
Author of *Got an Angry Kid? Parenting Spike, A Seriously Difficult Child*

"William Krill's book is greatly needed. PTSD is the most common aftermath of child abuse and often domestic abuse as well. There is a critical scarcity of mental-health professionals who know how to recognize child abuse, let alone treat it. The same goes for PTSD. I am relieved that someone is filling this gaping void."

—Fr. Heyward B. Ewart, III, Ph.D.
St. James the Elder Theological Seminary

Gentling

A Practical Guide to Treating
PTSD in Abused Children

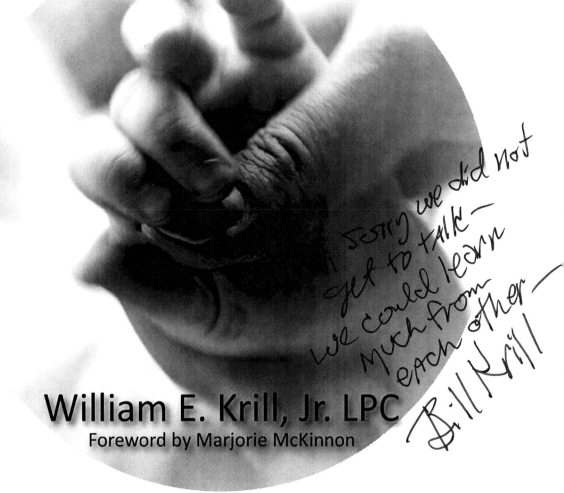

sorry we did not get to talk — we could learn much from each other —

Bill Krill

William E. Krill, Jr. LPC
Foreword by Marjorie McKinnon

New Horizons in Therapy Series
Loving Healing Press

Gentling: A Practical Guide to Treating PTSD in Abused Children
Copyright © 2010 William E. Krill, Jr. M.S.P.C. All Rights Reserved.
From the New Horizons in Therapy Series

Cover photo: W.A. Krill / Fighting Chance Photography

Library of Congress Cataloging-in-Publication Data

Krill, William E. (William Edwin), 1958-
  Gentling : a practical guide to treating PTSD in abused children / William E. Krill Jr.
    p. ; cm. -- (New horizons in therapy series)
  Includes bibliographical references and index.
  ISBN-13: 978-1-61599-003-0 (alk. paper)
  ISBN-10: 1-61599-003-8 (alk. paper)
  1. Post-traumatic stress disorder in children--Treatment. 2. Abused children--Mental health. I. Title. II. Series: New horizons in therapy series.
  [DNLM: 1. Stress Disorders, Post-Traumatic--therapy. 2. Child Abuse--therapy. 3. Child. 4. Empathy. 5. Professional-Patient Relations. WM 170 K925g 2019]
  RJ506.P55K75 2010
  618.92'8521--dc22
                          2009029692

Distributed by Ingram Book Group, Bertrams Books, New Leaf Distributing.

Published by
Loving Healing Press
5145 Pontiac Trail
Ann Arbor, MI 48105

www.LHPress.com
info@LHPress.com
Tollfree 888-761-6268
Fax 734-663-6861

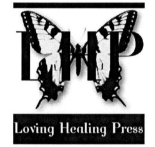

Contents

Foreword v

Introduction vii

Acknowledgements ix

1 – Gentling 1

2 – Trauma 3
    What is PTSD? 5
    PTSD and Children 6

3 – Signs and Symptoms Profile 9
    A Child Stress Profile 10
    Roger, Age 10 12
    Hallmarks of Stress.. 14

4 – Child-Specific Expressions of Stress Disorder Signs 19
    Physiological Signs.. 20
    Signs of Re-Experiencing 21
    Avoidance, Numbing and Detachment 23
    Relationship Confusion 25
    Trauma and Behavior Regression: A Case Study........................... 26
    Traumatic Stress and Memory 28
    Confusing Stress Behaviors with Common Childhood Behaviors ... 30

5 – Anatomy of the Stress Episode... 35

6 – A Course of Treatment for Abused Children with PTSD 41
    Treatment Objectives.. 42
    Gentling and emotive regulation 48

7 – Gentling and Treatment Objectives 51
    Lowering Physical and Psychological Agitation and Reactivity 51
    Helping the child to feel safe again 55
    Helping the child differentiate 58
    Self-Initiation of Learned Stress Reduction Techniques................ 60
    Resumption of Here and Now Development 63
    Experiencing of Positive Re-engagement.. 66

Reconnection, and Feeling Trust with Others 69
Approaching and Working Through the Critical Incident 72

8 – Problems with Traditional Behavior Modification Techniques 79
Angel, Age Seven 80

9 – Special Considerations in Sexual Trauma Cases 83

10 – An Environment of High Nurture, High Structure.........................87

11 – Helping to Break Negative Engagement Patterns 99

12 – Face-to-Face Gentling Countenance 103

13 – The Encopresis and Enuresis Problem 113
Educating Caregivers 114

14 – Stressed Self-Harm Management: Teaching Self-Comforting 119

15 – When the Child Begins to Share History......................................127
Rules for working with memory material of child victims......................129

16 – Understanding Secrets and Abuse 133

17 – When a Person is a Known Trigger 139

18 – The Family Preservation Bias 141
Educating Caregivers: Foster Parents, Teachers, CYS, and Judges.........141

19 – Stress Behavior Data Collection..145

20 – Classroom Protocols...151
[QT1] Suggestions to School Staff for a Stress Disordered Student) 154

21 – Self-Care for the Clinician or the Differentiated Helper 157

22 – Sample Treatment Plan...159

Postscript 161

Appendix A: Child Stress Profile 163

Appendix B: Handouts for Caregivers...169
[QT2] Caregiver's Instructions for Enuresis 169
[QT3] Caregiver's Instructions for Encopresis 171

Appendix "C" - Quick Teach Sheets..173
[QT4] Complex PTSD in Children..174
[QT5] False Accusations: Confabulation in Children with PTSD 176
[QT6] Encopresis and Enuresis in Stress Disordered Children................178
[QT7] Fostering a Sexually Abused Child 180
[QT8] How Acute Stress and PTSD Behavioral Signs May Be Confused With Normal Child Behaviors 183
[QT9] Stress Signs in Children with PTSD 186

[QT10] Recognizing Stress in Children 189
[QT11] Responding to a Highly Stressed Child 191
[QT12] Response Particulars to a Stress Disordered Child..........193
[QT13] Stress Inoculation for Children through Healthy Differentiation 197
What Is Stress Inoculation?...198
[QT14] Self-Harm Intervention 201
[QT15] The Course of Treatment for Children with PTSD 203
[QT16] Treating Episodes of Encopresis and Enuresis in Stress Disordered Children 205
[QT 17] When a Child Begins to Share Traumatic History 207

Appendix D: Stress Behavior Data Collection Forms............................209
Known Stress Behaviors...209
Stress Behavior Observation Log 210

About the Author..213

Bibliography 215

Index..223

Foreword

As a survivor of incest, while going through recovery, I read countless books on the subject. I attended retreats, seminars, watched video clips, listened to speakers and maneuvered my way through anything available to heal my soul from childhood sexual abuse. W. E. Krill's book, *Gentling : A Practical Guide to Treating PTSD in Abused Children*, intrigued me. If there is one term not yet included in any writing on child sexual abuse recovery it's "gentling." I had never given it much thought before, but as I read this page-turner I realized that the author was on to something unique that the rest of the world had neglected.

He grabbed me with his first sentence, "What would the world be like without gentleness?" Every page in this book touched a nerve, brought exhilaration. It was as if Mr. Krill knew exactly what goes on in the mind and the heart of a child sexual abuse victim.

He explains that the term PTSD was born after the Vietnam War, but over the years has changed to include victims from all walks of life, from young children to delayed-onset in our elders. His career has placed him in position to care for children who have been neglected, physically abused, sexually abused, and emotionally abused. As a result he has studied their behavior patterns, located the source and totality of their pain and decided on what they needed to heal. He points out that these children may spend years with the wrong diagnosis and ineffective treatment.

An abused child will not respond to pointed questions, to games directed at climbing inside their head, to "hints" that the clinician knows everything already. But they will respond to patience and gentling. The author says, "It is amazing to me how the child is sometimes the only one who "knows" what their diagnosis is".

This book, while directed at clinicians, should be read by anyone attempting to maneuver their way through the murky waters of child sexual abuse. It addresses every area of recovery with intelligence, sensitivity, and compassion. The innovative Child Stress Profile (CSP), and Quick Teach handouts such as "Fostering an Abused Child" and "Stress Signs in Children with PTSD," are just a few of the techniques the author utilizes. Mr. Krill's book is a jewel in the hands of anyone trying to heal, either themselves or others.

—Marjorie McKinnon,
Author of *REPAIR Your Life*, *REPAIR For Kids,* and *REPAIR For Toddlers*
Founder of *The Lamplighters*, a movement for recovery from incest and
childhood sexual abuse

Introduction

Like most books, this one has been long in the making. Not just the writing and publishing, but the roots of the book have been in formation for decades. The experiences of my life including my childhood, my education, my professional career, and those who have mentored and influenced me along the way, all played a part in this final fruit. Like the survivors that we mental health professionals treat, we are all the sum total of our life experiences, and our experiences, both good and bad cannot be forgotten or ignored.

The idea to write about the way that I approach and treat children who have had traumatic abuse events in their lives came to me a few years ago. I discovered that I perhaps was "on to something new" when others began to notice that I was having some success in relieving symptoms in children with PTSD. My search for specific approaches to small children only yielded articles describing the signs of trauma, and citations that "more study is needed" to test efficacy of various treatments. Most material concerning treatment described efforts with adult victims, and suggested adaptations of those methods to apply to children. While pre-adolescent and adolescent children may be approached more or less successfully with adapted adult methods, there remains no real articulated approach to young children suffering from stress disorders.

I cannot help but believe that there are countless clinicians out in the field that feel as frustrated as I did when I went searching for specific interventions and treatment plans to help these children. Since every recognized clinical approach needs to start somewhere, this book is an effort to put forth a practical approach to treatment of children with stress disorders. The approaches described are admittedly "untested" and a purely anecdotal account of what has worked for me. The method has developed largely by intuition as well as trial and error. The approach that I have developed has been largely intuitive. By paying close behavioral attention the children, they have taught me volumes.

In the past few years, I began to find that colleagues in the treatment of children were seeking me out to consult because I was becoming known as the guy who was having some success with stress disordered children. This forced me to consider how to articulate what it was that I was doing. This effort to organize the approach led me to produce one-page descriptions that I called "Quick Teach" sheets (see Appendix C) for fellow workers, including Behavior Specialists, Mobile Therapists, Therapeutic Support Staff, teachers, and foster parents. These became the seeds for this book.

Acknowledgements

My life, like yours, has intersected with people who have experienced terrible traumatic events. Most everyone we work with as clinicians have had some difficult if not traumatic events in their lives. Our friends and family have not been immune. Both my father and father-in-law served in World War II, and each bears the psychological and emotional effects of war.

Each have taught me through their relationship with me how a person is able to survive their experiences while effective treatment for Post Traumatic Stress was not even developed yet. Their willingness to share their stories with me has honored me. The children I work with daily are a constant reminder of the suffering that stress disorders create. When they come to trust me enough to share their stories, I am also honored.

There have been many teachers and healers who have influenced my clinical practice. I owe a great debt to all of the children who have allowed me the privilege to help them along their way in life. My heroes of healing have been people with a combination of gentleness, spirituality, assertiveness, and strength. The list includes people like Jean Vanier, Mother Teresa, Henri Nouwen, and Fred Rogers. My own parents raised me with a firm, kind gentleness that lives on through in my own parenting and work that I do daily with children.

I must give acknowledgement to Dr. Heide Sedwick, who has been a mentor, supporter, and cheerleader in my efforts with stress disordered children. At times I have felt that she has pumped up my ego far too much, as I know who real the "expert" in PTSD is. Her clinical direction, emotional support, and gentle but firm Franciscan supervision have motivated me to press ahead with this book.

<table>
<tr><td>1</td><td># Gentling</td><td>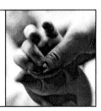</td></tr>
</table>

1 Gentling

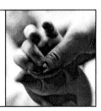

What would the world be like without gentleness? Gentleness is such a basic human characteristic that we often take it for granted. Gentleness appears to be so basic that even animals can be seen behaving in a gentle fashion following the birth of offspring. Some may argue that such behavior is simply instinctive for the animal mother; a measure to ensure the growth of the baby and thus the continuation of the species.

Certainly human beings bring *meaning* to what may be an instinctive behavior set. While gentleness may be instinctive, our experience of gentleness from others further teaches the subtleties of human kindness, and in turn, shapes how we are gentle with others. It would not be a stretch to say that a person's capacity for gentleness is an indication of civility; even a marker of what makes a human being *human* in the largest sense.

Hopefully, if the reader were to play a brief game of "word association", they would soon list the word "mother" or "father" in association with gentleness. And, what could be more nurturing than a parent's gentleness? Unfortunately, not all people are able to make this association so easily; their mother (or father) has not been gentle in their lives; they have experienced abuse and trauma at the hands of their loved ones.

Most people will also associate "healing" with gentleness, even though healing may involve some discomfort. Even when healing is not a possibility, there is gentleness to ease the discomfort of pain, and even the transition to death. "Gentling" is the process of delivering the balm of gentle gestures.

These gestures are complex and even at times may appear paradoxical: gentleness involves a kind of strength and assurance in the giver, and the gentleness may be delivered in a firm and assertive fashion. Of course, gentling also includes a calming countenance, a safe tone of voice sometimes paired with eyes filled with compassion, and an empathetic touch that can be as light as feather or as firm as a safe, encompassing hug.

Gentleness also may be easily associated with "spiritual". Most of the major religions of the world have an expression of their deity that is compassionate. As a person whose degree is in Pastoral Counseling, compassion is a core value of my vocation, how I help others, and why I do what I do. Even the secular clinician will recognize the value of using gentleness as a tool in their approach to helping others, and perhaps has even experienced the "miraculous" movement forward in a patient when they have had their empathic efforts accepted and used by the patient.

Though this approach has many familiar components that are certainly not new to the compassionate and caring helper, it is different because it uses these components in a very intentional, specific, and timely fashion. "Gentling" as a treatment for stress disordered children has its didactics and techniques, just like other approaches to helping children, but the foundation on which it is built is a firm and abiding faith in the power of gentleness and compassion. In a world where everything has a price, where the costs of violence are truly expensive, where hundreds of thousands of children each day face the harsh realities of traumatic events, gentleness is free.

2 Trauma

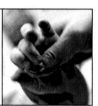

A trauma is an event that has happened to a person that has had a profound and life changing effect. The event may have resulted in the person having ongoing and uncomfortable symptoms. The symptoms might include re-experiencing (memories), avoidance, numbing, detachment, relationship problems, and alterations in the way that they view the world and physical symptoms that are similar to panic attacks.

Trauma affects everyone, either directly or indirectly. We all have people in our lives that have had difficult, and perhaps terrible things happen to them. Many times a day, we likely come into contact with people that we least expect to have had very traumatic experiences.

In recent months, I have come to learn more about a friend and colleague's life before I met her, and her life story could not be guessed from her current life. Each of us has had events in our own lives that have traumatized us and have caused us discomfort as a result. While one person's experience at having had a dog bite them may not be as dramatic or life-altering as a person who has survived a hurricane, torture, or rape, the process and discomfort are no less real.

Since trauma is all around us on a daily basis, and is what makes media headlines to catch viewers, it is easy to become numb to it. Certainly the "newsworthy" traumas beg for our attention, but there are countless private, quiet traumas that occur daily as well. On the nightly news we hear of young men and women who have died in the Global War on Terrorism, and see their grieving families.

Each day there are hundreds, if not thousands of children who are being neglected and abused in their families, by neighbors, strangers, or by the effects of war. Many of these children survive, for better or worse. Some do not survive. Sometimes survivors who gain healing go on to productive and happy lives, while others descend into lifelong pain, dysfunction, and may become perpetrators of trauma themselves.

Trauma always affects body, mind, emotions, and spirit. A person who has had a physical trauma, such as a motorcycle accident, will certainly have difficult emotions surrounding his or her misfortune. When a person is a victim of a psychological and emotional trauma, such as in the case of witnessing a loved one assaulted or abused, they may develop physical symptoms as a result of chemical changes in their body that occurred at the time of the assault. In situations where a child has been sexually abused, their body, mind, emotions, and spirit are altered and damaged. When viewed in this way, trauma can be seen for what it is: an all encompassing and profoundly life-altering disability.

To most of us, the reason why one person becomes symptomatic following a critical incident and the other does not is often a mystery. New research is beginning to demonstrate that in fact people who suffer symptoms for a long time after a trauma may have a brain chemistry that is prone to developing these symptoms. It does appear (and stands to reason, with their still developing brains) that young children may be more vulnerable to developing acute stress or posttraumatic stress.

Preconditions such as mental health disorders or high levels of everyday stress are also likely to be a factor. Children who live in marginal family situations with parents who have their own daily struggles to survive, or have mental health issues may also be more susceptible to developing symptoms. Children who, by circumstance, have poor "ego wrapping" may be more vulnerable to the effects of trauma and stress.

In families with intergenerational histories of domestic abuse, not only is abuse "inherited", but also stress disorders as well. However, the question of discerning the biophysical and genetic possibilities of connections between domestic abuse, child abuse, and PTSD are beyond the scope of this book.

Some children live in conditions with their biological families that are highly volatile, abusive, uncertain, and chaotic. These children may not have one single traumatic event that can be pinpointed as the source of their stress signs and symptoms. In their lives, the constant high level of stress may create behavioral effects in them that look very much like the ones seen in children who have survived other, more specific trauma. The diagnostic and treatment community needs to recognize and codify this kind of traumatic stress as just as valid as acute and post-traumatic stress. The story, sources, study, results, treatment and treatment outcomes of trauma are far from complete.

A child may suffer for many years without the proper diagnosis. In some cases, the critical incident(s) may be unknown to the adults around the child. In situations where the child has been sexually perpetrated upon, the child may be holding the secret quite closely. If the child is very young (age six or below), the trauma may have occurred at a time before memory was fully developed; even if they want to tell you about the trauma, they cannot recall enough details of the event or articulate what they are feeling.

In other situations, the adult caregivers simply do not connect the dots between the critical incident and the child's behaviors. This is especially true in chaotic families that have a long history of domestic violence and varieties of abuse. In these families, the child's behaviors are the norm, and the family only becomes aware of a problem when the child enters school.

What is PTSD?

The rudiments of a modern understanding of PTSD are reflected in the medical literature as early as the American Civil War, when surgeon Jacob Mendes Da Costa identified what came to be called 'soldier's heart', a grouping of symptoms that looked like heart disease, but revealed no physiological abnormalities of heart problems. It came to be understood in the medical field as a grouping of symptoms indicating a severe anxiety reaction associated with battle experience.

By the time of World War I, the popular label for PTSD becomes "shell shock", a reasonable description considering the heavy artillery barrages of that war. Films from the era show soldiers in states of dissociation or uncontrolled trembling, as well as cases of apparent leg and arm paralysis, or sudden, unexplained blindness. In World War II, "battle fatigue" became the phrase for the collection of signs and symptoms. The disorder was still highly misunderstood by most lay people, with soldiers continuing associate the symptoms as a proof of being a 'coward', a word that carried much weight for soldiers of that day. Subsequent examination and research of the Holocaust survivors of Nazi concentration camps and the bombing survivors of throughout Europe and Japan revealed extremely similar effects on non-combatants. Not much progress on the issue appears to have been made during the Korean War years.

Many courageous but damaged veterans of the Viet Nam War pressed the mental health community (not to mention the US government) into consideration of the symptom and behavioral sign clusters as something more than a simple and passing anxiety or adjustment to post-battle life. The psychological community traditionally formulates new or adapted diagnoses as a result of a large body of clinical experience, and this appears to be the case for the eventual formulation of 'PTSD' first introduced in the Diagnostic Statistics Manual III (DSM-III) in 1980. It certainly can be argued that there may have been significant political forces at work as to why it took so long after Viet Nam to recognize PTSD, but that is beyond the scope of the present work.

Interestingly, even anecdotal accounts of war-related PTSD symptoms appear to have differences in expression throughout the previously discussed wars, suggesting that present culture may greatly impact the expression of the symptoms and signs of the disorder. It would appear that our understandings of PTSD are still in a stage of adolescence, and are not yet fully mature. I have certainly come to the conclusion that child abuse victims have their own unique expression of PTSD.

The progress of mental health care, treatment, and early intervention in the past thirty years has come to recognize that it is not just war veterans who can develop painful signs and symptoms. Police officers, firefighters, victims of natural disasters, victims of domestic abuse and crime can all suffer from posttraumatic stress. In particular, the last ten to fifteen years of recognition, research, and treatment expansion for stress disorders has progressed significantly.

Indeed, the controversy in the mental health community over the PTSD diagnosis continues with suggestions that developmental trauma (abuse), though not having one single point of critical incident, qualifies for a PTSD diagnosis.

It is likely that any human being, when exposed long enough to repeated critical incidents, will take on a classic acute or posttraumatic stress profile of behaviors. Furthermore, I believe that any person, at any time, may become acutely reactive if an incident occurs at an emotionally vulnerable time and the event has emotional value to them. While the event and circumstance may not be evident to the observer as traumatic, it is the subjective experience that counts the most. We are all vulnerable.

PTSD and Children

Anyone who works closely with victims can tell you how contagious the stress is. Even the most experienced clinicians will experience an emotional toll, have intrusive dream content, and have moments in treatment when they become overwhelmed with grief, fear, and deep sadness (secondary PTSD). Part of the clinician's job is to remember to take care of themselves as well as the victim. I use the word 'victim' rather than 'survivor' because abused children *are* victims of a crime, and the effects of PTSD, left under and untreated, continue to *keep* them victims for years, even decades. For many, time is a second perpetrator. A child can only become a survivor when someone recognizes their PTSD and has effective means to begin to help them to heal.

My career has placed me in position to care for children who have been neglected, physically abused, sexually abused, and emotionally abused. Many of these children have been removed from their families and live with foster parents, who struggle to care for them despite the behavioral effects of posttraumatic stress. My experience with children has led me to understand that children have their own unique behavioral expressions that do not necessarily match the adult victim's behaviors. As such, many children with Acute Stress Disorder or PTSD may spend years with the wrong diagnosis and ineffective treatment.

Just as in the treatment of physical trauma, both immediate treatment and long-term rehabilitation are needed in psychological trauma. The healing process is not always comfortable, and the healer may need to help the patient tolerate the discomfort of treatment through encouragement and gentle nursing. While some pain is expected and perhaps even necessary for healing, the overriding key to stress disorder treatment in children is the application of the balm of gentleness.

Children, in fact, may experience trauma differently than adults do, and so then the treatment may also call for a different approach than what is used for adults. Adults who experience their critical event as adults naturally have much more history behind them and many more positive healthy ego experiences. As such, the adult survivor has a "well of resources" to draw from in order to begin to make sense of their traumatic event. They have the ability to make comparisons of their life before the events as opposed to after the event.

Small children who have experienced chaotic lives and multiple traumas since birth have no such wellspring to draw from. A child who has lived their entire life in the midst of a war, for example, has nothing to compare their experience to; no safe and comforting memory to retreat to when the time comes that they need to "go somewhere else" in their head to escape the intensity of the moment.

In traditional adult treatment of trauma, the patient is strongly encouraged to get right to the processing of the traumatic events and memories. The adult is encouraged to detail the events and articulate their corresponding emotions. This process may also be effective when used with a child of adolescent age. It can be assumed that the adult or adolescent has a fair understanding and ability to quickly develop trust in the clinician as a helper.

The idea of "counselor" is quite ingrained in most cultures as a positive concept. But what if the child is five or six years old, has an intellectual disability, and has a severe speech impediment? Or what if the child has had multiple adult perpetrators of violence against them?

Young children often have difficulty in articulating their experiences effectively, even if they are not traumatic experiences. Their self-awareness of internal processes is extremely limited, not because of their trauma, but simply because of their developmental stage. It becomes obvious that the treatment approaches for adults and teens becomes awkward at best when applied to young children.

Traumatic *stress reactivity* is a disease. The definition of a disease is something that affects the body that is destructive and progressive. Left untreated, many victims indeed get worse.

When too many critical incidents or stress reactivity episodes happen, the victim gets pushed over the edge to a realm of mental health disorder that they cannot easily come back from. Those who decide to cope with drugs and alcohol begin to suffer the effects from such abuse, including death. Victims of physical or sexual trauma may begin to live lifestyles that ensure their continued victimization. People can die in any number of ways due to their history of traumatic events.

Some lucky few victims of trauma happen upon ways to heal themselves. These lucky few are victims that have a solid history of an adequate "ego wrapping". In the case of soldiers, such as my own father, they may have among their resources an intensely strong faith life that acted as their "lifesaver." Or, as in the case of my father-in-law, an extremely sharp and intense intellect kept it at bay.

Both of these fine men also had the unshakable knowledge that there were loved ones that were ready and willing to provide them with the support and affection that they would need to heal when they returned home. But even in these cases, there are residual signs and symptoms that are clearly scars that still ache.

The young child who finds himself suddenly in a foster home following the five years of his (entire) life spent in a trailer that doubled as a meth lab, neglected, physically and sexually abused is at a considerably greater disadvantage. Next, I'll proceed to articulate how a clinician might take on the daunting task of trying to help this child.

3 Signs and Symptoms Profile

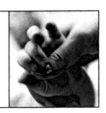

The treating psychologist hands you a diagnosis: Post Traumatic Stress Disorder. Now what? Most clinicians will begin to take a closer look at the child's behaviors. What does the parent or foster parent say the child is doing? What treatment has been tried in the recent past? What worked, what did not?

In many cases, clinicians inherit PTSD cases from other clinicians. The sad fact is there are not enough well-trained clinicians who understand stress disorders, let alone stress disorders in children. I have received cases that have been in services for years and years, having had many therapists, and yet with no real discernable progress.

In review of the case file and past treatment plans, I often find that the clinician attacked the behavior problems in what might be termed a very generic fashion. The goals often center on "ending tantrums", "learning anger management techniques", or "gaining better social skills." While all of these areas may be important and valid, they often are not a sharp enough focus for children with a PTSD diagnosis. These areas are what I call "wide brushstrokes" of behaviors. The stress-disordered child needs a finer and more precise brush stroke in their treatment approach.

In a later chapter, I will outline a sample treatment plan. But for now, it is important to lay the groundwork for that plan. As alluded to earlier, each person has his or her own unique and subjective experience of a traumatic event. So too, each person has more or less a very individualized demonstration of their distress. While we can certainly make generalizations of signs and symptoms common to most victims, each victim will have a personal profile of signs and symptoms. This information has very important implications in treatment for several reasons.

First, when the clinician can accurately assess which behavioral signs and symptoms that the victim has, there develops a baseline view of behaviors that can be compared to later for improvements in treatment. Secondly, this data can help to focus the areas of treatment, and create a protocol of what behavioral areas to treat first, second, and so on. Next, this information can be used directly with the victim to help sensitize them to the processes that go on inside their body and the behaviors that they engage in.

In many cases, children have lived so long with their stress behaviors; they do not even realize that they are abnormal. In addition, this list of signs and symptoms can be used to educate all of the adults in the child's life, such as parents, foster parents, teachers, therapeutic support staff, guidance counselors, ministers, lawyers, and judges. In cases where legal issues related to abuse are present, such clinical behavioral data becomes very important in demonstrating if and when the child is ready to return to their biological family.

A Child Stress Profile

In my clinical experience, I have noticed that children, while having many of the behavioral signs well-documented in adult PTSD victims, have either different expressions of these signs, or have unique signs only seen in children. Behavioral stress signs in children can range from quite dramatic to very subtle. A Stress Profile can help the clinician recognize some of these unique expressions as sourced in stress signs and not some other area. A brief example of this would be the common assessment that a child is behaving in an "oppositional" manner, when in fact; they may be expressing defensive behaviors related to a trauma memory.

Gaining the ability to differentiate when a set of behaviors has its source in a traumatic event in history rather than a child simply misbehaving or demonstrating a "tantrum" is important in the daily care of the child. When pressure is applied to the (apparently oppositional) child with PTSD, the child's difficult behaviors often increase rather than decrease. Truly oppositional children will comply with pressure at some point. It is also important to the long term goal of easing the behavioral effects of PTSD, because when a child is given ordinary discipline to control PTSD behaviors, the PTSD behaviors are driven deeper, making them harder to treat.

The taking of a Child Stress Profile (CSP) should not be confused with an "assessment". An assessment leads to a diagnosis, and is completed by a psychologist. The CSP is a tool that a clinician uses following the diagnosis to begin to gain a clear picture of the child's stress related behaviors.

This becomes particularly important if the child has other issues that affect their behaviors, such a co-morbid mental health condition, or have lived in a household with inadequate discipline. Lots of children have had their stress symptoms confused with their lack of discipline. When the former is treated as if it were the latter, neither condition improves.

I developed the Child Stress Profile out of my desire to better understand, organize, and measure children's stress behaviors and treatment outcomes. After having used it for two years, I was pleased to see that it demonstrated clear progress in the children I was treating. The CSP uses six sub-scales (or categories) of signs and symptoms, including the three classic symptom areas drawn from the DSM-IV: re-experiencing, avoidance-numbing-detachment, and psychobiological alterations.

The other three categories (personal relationships, psychological alterations, and self structure) have been taken from *Treating Psychological Trauma & PTSD* (Wilson, Friedman, and Lindy, 2001). Specific signs and symptoms were gleaned both from the DSM-IV and the work of Wilson, Freidman, and Lindy. I have placed a "spin" on many items so that they more accurately reflect what I have seen in children. Some items are the result of my own clinical experience of signs and symptoms common to children with stress disorders.

The resulting Child Stress Profile (CSP) tool has just over 100 items contained in six different sub-scales. The tool is designed for the clinician to conduct an interview with significant adults in the child's life, preferably caretakers. If more than one person is being interviewed at the same time, I use a consensus method to determine the most accurate response. The interviewing clinician may need to give some further explanation for some of the items by giving examples, etc. When completed, the clinician scores the responses.

Please turn to the Appendix A of this book to review the actual questions contained in the CSP. The scoring block is reproduced below:

SCORING: Indicate the number of each response in each grouping

Range	Sub-scale	D	FN	NI	FI
Items 1-27	Allostatic process and load (27)				
Items 28-44	Re-experience (17)				
Items 45-60	Avoidance, numbing & detachment (16)				
Items 61-72	Personal relationships (12)				
Items 73-90	Psychological alterations (18)				
Items 91-102	Self structure (12)				
	Totals				

Scoring the CSP is not difficult. The number of each response for each symptom grouping is tallied and recorded. The balance or percentage of items in the 'intense' range then can be discerned, along with the balance between 'not frequent, but intense' and 'frequent and intense'.

Interpreting results is also quite simple; in most cases where the child has a PTSD diagnosis the initial Profile scores for each area will have above or about 50% of the responses in the "intense" range. For example, if the child has a PTSD diagnosis, then sum of NI and FI marked questions in through items 45-60, then he or she will probably score 9 or higher (above 50%).

It is important to note that the Child Stress Profile is not intended to be a scientific/statistical instrument, but a practical, clinical 'profile' descriptor of the individual's unique symptom status; a snapshot in time. It is not intended to compare one survivor to another (or a group of others), but a tool for understanding the individual. The idea is that the clinician uses the tool as an outcomes measure to keep track of the lowering of symptoms from 'frequent and intense' to 'not frequent, but intense, to 'frequent, but not intense' to near cessation of negative impact on the individual.

Generally, stress disordered children score in the mid 50-60% in the 'intense' range (total score) then drop below the 50% and lower as treatment progresses. The Profile is repeated approximately every three to four months in treatment to test outcomes and direct treatment focus. If a child scores well below 50% in the allostatic process and load category (for example, having only six items in the 'intense' range), then consideration of a different diagnosis would be in order.

Adaptations must be made when using the CSP for very small children under the age of five. They, of course will not be able to give any accurate indications on items such as self-esteem or guilt expressions, though these may be somewhat apparent to the observer being interviewed through the child's behaviors and expressions. In cases where an opinion of the observer cannot be formed, I simply score the child as "D" for that particular item. The following case example will provide the reader with clearer understanding of how the Child Stress Profile can be used for both treatment focus and as an outcomes measure.

Roger, Age 10

I began to work with Roger several years ago when he had just turned ten years old and had been in his foster home for a few months. He had been removed from his family by the county child protective services following a report from local police that they had found Roger tied to a railing on a second story balcony of the family home and was being beaten by his seventeen year old sister who had been left in charge of him. The only parent in the home, the children's mother, could not be located, and the children did not know where the mother was. It was later discovered that she had been at local club and was intoxicated.

Subsequent investigation revealed that the sanitary conditions in the home were barely acceptable, and the child protective services had multiple reports in the past year of the children being neglected and totally unsupervised. The mother had mental health issues of her own, impressing either as an untreated bi-polar or a borderline personality. Within a few months of being in the foster home, Roger had further revealed to the county worker that he had been sexually abused by his mother's former paramour. A bright, sensitive, and kindly boy, Roger clearly loved and was concerned about his mother, and held very strong anger for his sister and the mother's paramour.

Using the Child Stress Profile with the foster parents yielded an initial score of 62% of items in the intense range, with the larger percentage of items in the 'frequent and intense' category. He had 21 items in the 'intense' range in the allostatic load and process category, as would be expected with his PTSD diagnosis and history of critical incidents. He had consecutively, 10 items in the intense range for re-experiencing, 10 items in avoidance, numbing and detachment, with 9 items in psychological alterations, 7 items in the personal relationships, and 6 in self structure.

The immediate challenge was to begin to lower Roger's high reactivity to cues and triggers. To do this, the foster parents were given a list of the items that Roger scored in the intense range on the CSP and were asked to be extra observant of him for several weeks to ascertain any possible cues that could be discerned. In addition, they were also educated concerning the Gentling base philosophy and techniques for early intervention in the allostatic process and the approaches for de-escalating those stress episodes that started. It was important that Roger gain a sense of safety and security in the foster home as quickly as possible in order to begin to educate him on his own behavioral signs and symptoms as well as a means to interrupt these on his own.

The school was contacted, and I gained access to the classroom to observe Roger at school. The teacher reported that he did well in all academic and social areas, but tended to slack off for days at a time. She also noted that these seemed to correspond to the visits he had with his biological mother. He expressed his stress with behaviors well within the CSP category descriptions. In school, he would often appear to be daydreaming or lackadaisical, but also demonstrated signs of numbing when he interacted with peers. He would often roughhouse with other boys, but seemed to become too aggressive and have no empathy when they got hurt. On the flip side, he was hypersensitive and reactive to others even slightly injuring him.

In the foster home, Roger had frequent nightmares, but could not or would not discuss them. In addition, he had almost nightly wetting, despite the foster parents limiting drinks after dinner and the use of a prescription medication to alleviate the problem. He also displayed many of the same peer interaction problems seen in school with the other children in the foster home, but less so with the foster family's biological children, who were a bit older and had experience with foster children in the past.

Roger was able to form a fairly rapid trust with me, and began to take interest in learning about his own stress related behaviors due to the embarrassment he had over wetting the bed and being inconsistent in his peer relationships. Fortunately, he had a sparkling personality that when not stressed, was also charming and entertaining. He was quite frustrated at gaining new friends only to distance them when he began to have stress episodes. The result of his motivation for change was that he began to work hard at altering his basic daily stress levels through recognition of his cues and triggers, as well as learning a bit about self calming techniques through the use of a portable Galvanic Skin Resistance monitor I use just for that purpose. Most children are fascinated by the GSR, and find it a challenge to 'change the sound' that it emits by relaxing. With children who are curious and bright the GSR can produce rapid results in the child's understanding of their physiological stress signs and signs of relaxation.

In addition to work on the physical aspects of his stress reactivity, we also began work on how to manage the material that was intruding on his dreams, and began to offer him skills to practice in the foster home; allowing the foster parents to coach him. Often, this work was done in the presence of the foster parents, as a means not only to transfer skills to them, but foster the security, safety, and attachment that is so very supportive of recovery.

As a result, within six months, Roger's CSP percentages were dropping significantly, and continued to drop throughout the two and half years of treatment; about 15% a year, until I exited the case with a satisfying overall score on the CPS of 30% of items in the intense range. It should be noted though, there were setbacks reflected in the three month re-evaluations of the CPS, most notably when Roger 's custody issues were reviewed in court twice a year; Roger became very anxious about the possibility that he may have to return to his mother's home. One major intervention during the last six months of my treatment with him that I believe helped him to overcome these anxieties was when he asked if it would be all right if he wrote a letter to his mother to tell he about how angry he was with her. While I fully supported the letter writing, I also assured Roger that he should only send the letter after he had 'slept on it' for a few days. While he ultimately did not send the letter, writing it gave him what he needed to later confront her in a calm, dignified, and respectful manner that further advanced his healing.

Hallmarks of Stress

If the reader is relatively new to working with children who have been diagnosed with Acute Stress or Post Traumatic Stress, they need to become familiar with the six basic groupings of signs and symptoms that the Profile uses. Characteristically, the first grouping, allostatic process and load, is the hallmark of stress disorders and will score fairly high in most cases. There will be a unique combination of scores for the other five areas for each child with a stress disorder, with the possibility of some fairly low scores in a particular symptom grouping (below 50% of the total in the 'intense' range. A high score in the allostatic load and process category with a low score in self structure and psychological alterations gives the clinician a clue as to the child's strengths and less damaged areas that can then be used to build a treatment strategy upon.

Allostasis is our body's way of trying to stay stable during stressful events. For example, when the traffic light turns yellow, I have a moment of increased stress: should I brake, or accelerate? The event adds just a bit of stress load to my already busy day, but I am likely to be able to continue to manage it.

When a person has a high stress critical incident, his or her body and mind have to work overtime in order to absorb and cope with the insult. If the person has multiple critical incidents over a relatively short period of time, or suffers through intermittent, unpredictable critical incidents, then the body, mind, emotional, and behavioral reactions can become quite complex. The victim can come to a point where they are bearing a very high allostatic load. The allostatic processes in their body are complex and negatively impact their behavior and daily life.

The body of a person who has lived through critical incidents learns allostatic processes. When under a high level of stress, many chemicals flood into the bloodstream in order to motivate the person to do what is needed to preserve their life. Fear is a very primal motivator, and in most cases, the response will either be fight-or-flight. The fight-or-flight (allostatic process) reaction kicks in with lightning speed when the victim experiences a cue or trigger in the world around them. Cues and triggers are things in the environment that remind (consciously or unconsciously) the victim of a traumatic event.

For those readers, like myself, who have not had Acute Stress (AS) or PTSD, an admittedly pale analog of the process that goes on inside the body of a PTSD victim would be to picture yourself going for a ride on a rollercoaster: prior to getting on the rollercoaster, your body is already under the stress of anticipation. It increases when you board the train, and heightens further just at the top of the big hill. You may want to appear courageous, only to let loose a scream on the downhill.

Now, if you have been on this particular rollercoaster several times, your body may get used to the higher level of stress and it will seem far less intense. This comparison really only works if you are a person who does not enjoy rollercoasters. Those people who hate rollercoasters can become very uncomfortable even viewing one or talking about one. Those who enjoy rollercoasters have been able to reconcile the physical allostatic load with mindful thoughts that they are completely safe.

The above description is a very, very simplistic comparison of what a victim goes through. The allostatic load, processes, and resultant symptoms and behaviors that they suffer are complex, disabling, and painful. But the good news is that if a person's body has learned reactions to perceived threats, then their body can also learn to perceive things in a new way, and change uncontrolled reactions to considered responses to the cues and triggers that they find all around them.

We all "re-experience" memories every day, so re-experiencing is not an especially strange experience. When we look at a photograph of a loved one, we will likely recall the event where the photo was taken, and revisit in a very real way the emotions we have for the person in the picture. The photograph is physical cue that triggers a specific memory and set of emotions.

When a stress disordered person perceives a cue in the world around them that reminds them of a traumatic event in their past, they may begin to re-experience the trauma as a vivid memory that elicits all of the emotions and physical reactions that they originally experienced. While some people still use the term "flashback" to describe this, that term has many connotations with the LSD users and so "re-experience" is a more accurate term. Another significant re-experiencing effect is sleep disturbance and nightmares. While at the edge of sleep, the ego is very vulnerable to intrusive thoughts and memories. Nightmares seem to be a prevalent experience of victims, and are especially disturbing to children.

Once again, the reader will be able to relate to the next grouping of signs and symptoms: avoidance, numbing, and detachment. Most everyone has had an experience of avoiding a person, place, or thing they find unpleasant. The experience of emotional numbness is familiar to anyone who has someone they love die, as is the feeling of detachment we may feel when we are estranged from someone important in our lives.

The person who suffers from a stress disorder feels all of these things, but much more intensely and consistently than the average person. In the average person, these emotions fade over time. For the victim of PTSD, they may be a daily occurrence for many years.

Due to the first three groupings of symptoms, it is not surprising that the personal relationships of people with stress disorders become disrupted. Those who live with, or in the case of children, care for AS or PTSD victims often become very frustrated and desperate in their relationships with them. Trust and intimacy for an AS or PTSD victim become central issues in their relationships. A victim's behaviors are often unpredictable, confusing, and even violent. In the case of adults with stress disorders, they often have a long string of broken relationships. For children with the disorder, they struggle to continue a normal social development.

Following a critical incident or multiple traumas, most people have their view of the world altered in some way. The way they begin to think of the world around them, their basic psychological makeup, may be altered to some degree. Certainly the wide community experience of 9-11 has altered not only individual psychology, but the entire nations.

When personal relationships and psychological makeup are altered, the individual's self-concept and how they structure the self will also be impacted. Anyone who has had a loved one go off to war and return will tell you about the fundamental change that took place in the person. Many people who survived hurricane Katrina have had their relationships and self-concept changed forever.

Trauma profoundly affects how an individual restructures the essence of who they are in order to make sense of the trauma and the world around them; this is done in order to survive. The restructuring can result in difficult and uncomfortable symptoms, or, the restructuring can result in an individual who has moved through their trauma, and has become a person who can once again grow and love life.

In the next section, some details of the behavioral signs of traumatic stress reactivity will be explored in more thorough manner to help the clinician conduct the Child Stress Profile interview in the most effective manner possible.

4 Child-Specific Expressions of Stress Disorder Signs

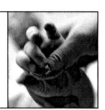

The dual challenge is to first understand the signs and symptoms that are specific to children with PTSD, and then those signs and symptoms specific to one particular child. As mentioned earlier, in my clinical experience, children, especially young children, seem to have behavioral expressions of stress disorder that look different than those of adults with stress disorder. At first glance, the broad strokes of symptom identification, such as the six large grouping of signs, looks pretty much the same. But when individual expressions or discrete behaviors are observed, children will have behaviors that adults generally do not have, or rarely have. The six areas of behavioral stress disorder signs need to be viewed through the developmental level that the child is at.

It is almost axiomatic that children will have some quantity or quality differences in behavioral expressions than adults do, even when both share the same mental health disorder. A stark example of the behavioral differences between adults and children is the fact that the majority of stress disorder cases that I have dealt with in very young children have all had wetting/soiling issues (beyond the potty learning age) that have not responded to the usual forms of therapeutic intervention. In many of these cases, the child not only is encopretic (involuntary defecation not attributable to physical defects or illness) , but also engages in feces manipulation or smearing.

Children's behavioral expressions of stress disorder are complicated by the fact that they are children: many adults will chalk up the behaviors that they see as other, more common childhood behaviors such as stubbornness, being spoiled, or "tantrums". Each of these behaviors, when viewed through the lens of PTSD and the perspective of developmental limitations, transform into something a bit more complicated. Indeed, one of the telling signs that a child may be suffering from PTSD is that the ordinary applications of guidance and discipline (not to mention medication) do not seem to be effective.

In addition, the child's relative level of development in all spheres must also be taken into consideration; what may appear to be a severely immature child may be a child who once had near age-appropriate maturity, but now is experiencing regressions due to trauma. The child's basic developmental level appears to have impact on the behavioral signs, especially those signs that have to do with ego cohesion. The younger the child, the less primary, healthy ego development they have gained prior to the trauma.

Physiological Signs

Physiological changes in the child's body following trauma (allostatic process) are likely essentially the same as in an adult's body, but the behavioral expressions may easily be confused with other disorders than acute stress or PTSD. In adult cases of PTSD, there is generally a very good understanding that the person had some dramatic behavioral changes following a traumatic event, such as battle. With PTSD cases in children, the behaviors are often confused with tantrums or other mental health diagnoses.

Often, children demonstrate very rapid onset of physical and emotional agitation with equally rapid change back to relative calmness. Caretakers and clinicians will describe this effect as a "light switch". One moment, the child will be calm and happy, the next moment extremely upset and inconsolable, or agitated and aggressive.

This is followed by a rather rapid calming and the child "switching back" to a happy child. Also, the child may appear to have little memory about the upset or what caused it. Another pattern seems to be that the child becomes physically and emotionally agitated, with "waves" of upset, and may stay that way for extended periods of time (hours or days.)

This may be followed once again by a relatively calm period of days or weeks. It is easy to see how one might think that the child may have Attention-Deficit Hyperactivity Disorder (ADHD) or bi-polar disorder. Misdiagnosis may be due to the psychologist not receiving the information needed concerning a specific trauma event to make them aware of a stress disorder possibility. The parent of the child may conveniently forget the important event, or, the family may have a long history of multiple, smaller stressors that are simply taken as non-sequitur in their lives.

A fairly typical stress episode seen in young children with PTSD follows a pattern such as this: either an internal or external cue triggers the biological reaction, the child begins to escalate in emotional and physical agitation, the stress peaks, and then the child reaches a point of exhaustion that may proceed either to tears, sleep, or a very rapid "light switch" return to normalcy. The whole process may be only a matter of moments, or it may be a process that takes hours. In my observation, a child tends to have a fairly predictable pattern of activation and movement through a stress episode that is unique to the individual.

Close observation of the child will reveal early, subtle clues that the child's stress level is building. A good place to start is to ask the caregiver if they can spot an upset brewing, and what it is they exactly see that tells them so. During the stress episode, the clinician should pay close attention to the physiological demonstrations that the child is presenting.

Many children will present with a variety of signs, including generalized physical agitation, flat affect, flushed cheeks, pupil dilation, body rigidity, vocal changes (guttural or animal like sounds, or high pitched screams, or even complete silence). There may be hiding behaviors (under tables, desks, closets), or running away behaviors. In cases of sexual trauma history, there may be sexually precocious behavior, such as use of words and expressions uncommon to a child of a particular age.

There may be over-friendly physical expressions such as hugs and caresses that feel "creepy" to the adult. There may be spontaneous release of bladder and bowel in extreme cases. In milder cases, the child may complain of feeling ill, such as about to vomit. The point of this observation and recording of the child's specific and unique pattern of stress indicators is not only to enable highly target treatment for each behavior later on, but to become better at spotting the child's building stress, and possible longer term rhythms of symptom presentation. Understanding the particular child's particular stress tolerance and any longer term patterns of exacerbation are keys to interrupting an episode before it occurs.

In witnessing many stress episodes in children diagnosed with PTSD, perhaps the sign with the most impact on me has been the clear sense that the child is "not with me". During stress episodes, there is a clear sense the child is in a dissociative state to some degree. This effect can be quite mild and last only a few moments, or it can be very intense and last hours.

When the effect is intense, the child may demonstrate signs such as speaking gibberish to themselves, curling up in a fetal position, taking their clothes off, sexual self-stimulation, and have rapid eye darting. There is quite often an extremely flat affect and glassy eyes with pupil dilation. The important thing for the clinician to remember is that each child will have a unique, particular Stress Profile of physical reactivity behaviors.

Signs of Re-Experiencing

Re-experiences of a critical incident can vary in intensity and duration. Re-experiencing can range from the child recalling memories with no emotion, appropriate emotion, or all-out rage. As mentioned earlier concerning allostatic signs, children may clearly dissociate during re-experiencing events.

This can look like simple "daydreaming" or be more intense with glassy eyes and extreme fear presenting. The child may also be engaged in play activities with dolls or action figures that becomes oddly intense and includes dialogs that sound decidedly grown up. If an adult tries to interrupt the re-enactment play, the child may respond as if deaf.

Re-experiencing behavioral signs can also include the child becoming panicky, running away, and hiding. If the child is recalling an assault in their past, they will essentially either defend themselves with fight or flight as they did during the assault. One small girl in my care, who was suspected of having been sexually abused by her mother's paramour, was playing nicely with me coloring in a coloring book, when she suddenly became quite agitated, jumped up, and threw herself on the blow-up toy clown punching bag nearby. She began to scream, "Get off me, you bastard!" and moan in decidedly sexual manner at the same time. This spooky feeling episode (for me) illustrated a clear re-experiencing for the child, and gave me some clues that perhaps it was not she herself who had been sexually assaulted, but her mother, in her presence.

When an adult challenges PTSD children for even relatively minor misbehavior, they can be seen sometimes reacting like a deer caught in the headlights. This "freezing" effect may be accompanied by clear expressions of fear, including flinching, eye contact avoidance, or flat affect. Even when adults (such as teachers) apply the normative pressure to a child to comply with a directive or to complete schoolwork, the stress-disordered child may be triggered into a re-experience of pressure they felt during their abuse trauma.

The teacher, not understanding the child's issue, and seeing "oppositional behavior" naturally applies more pressure to the child. If the child were truly simply defiant, they would comply at some point during the pressure. But the stress-disordered child is now in a re-experience situation where they are overreacting and mistakenly reacting; they are defending themselves from perceived harm from yet another possible abuse situation.

Close observation of the child's play will also often give examples of re-experience. Play skills are often underdeveloped: there may be intolerance for individual play, parallel play quickly becomes intrusive to other children, and cooperative play is disturbed. Lack of sharing or grabbing toys may be seen. The play is likely to be at least bossy, if not aggressive and violent. Stress Disordered children spend a good bit of recess time standing in the time-out section of the playground. Play with particular toys such as dollhouses or action-figures are often excessively violent or precocious, with the child consistently undressing the dolls.

There are some theories that the play re-enactments are the efforts of the child to process their trauma. While this may be true, excessive re-enactment play may lead to behavioral problems when re-enactments with toys transition to re-enactments with other children. The clinician has a duty not only to explore and vent the violent history and attempt to heal the child from their horrible memories, but to help shape the child's play by demonstrating and engaging the child in more age normative, appropriate play.

Avoidance, Numbing and Detachment

Avoidance, numbing, and detachment in young children also follows a predictable pattern, that while paralleling adult expressions, may not be interpreted by adults correctly, or presents differently. Stress disordered children, if they are in foster care, or do not have contact with their perpetrator, will seem at times to have forgotten all about their "former" lives. In this respect, children do what adults do: they actively avoid any references to the painful past.

The difference seems to be that the child will often totally ignore and not respond at all to any mention of the past or the trauma. It is almost as if they become deaf when a person, place, or item is mentioned connected with the trauma. This effect may of course, be due in some varying part to the fact that many perpetrators give stern warnings and threats to children to keep quiet about the abuse/critical incidents.

A curious and startling effect of numbing in abused children is that they will often demonstrate a marked lack of distress or pain when injured in a way that would leave most children screaming. Sound bumps on the head, falls, and bloody skinned knees may give rise only to a momentary pause in play. On the other hand, they also may become disconsolate over very small injuries that other children would simply shake off. Because of the physiological issues of stress, these reactions may be closely connected to the allostatic process.

If the child's body operates at a very high level of stress most of the time, their pain tolerance may be altered as if in a state of perpetual shock. This effect can be seen in combat, when soldiers are able to continue to fight in desperate situations even though they are severely wounded. The wound, at any other time agonizing, is numb for the time being.

Foster parents, in particular have noted that children diagnosed with PTSD have a high rate of variable attachment. There appears to be a wide continuum of attachment and detachment that may also have a unique pattern to the individual child. The child may be very affectionate, caring, and clingy one moment, and cold, rejecting, or totally detached the next.

This attachment and detachment continuum has implications with all of the child's relationships and potential relationships. While some children quickly become overly-familiar with strangers, other children will avoid new people with determination. The overly friendly children can be misinterpreted as simply being a friendly child, and the avoidant child as being shy. Each has a social liability. The overly friendly child may be vulnerable to re-victimization, and the avoidant child may become delayed in social isolation.

Both strategies of the children clearly have wisdom. The overly friendly child may be trying to seek adult protection (or the strategy is to try to please a potential angry perpetrator.) The avoidant child is simply trying to be very sure that the new person is safe.

The clinician may be aware that one of the Rule Out diagnoses common in association with PTSD in children is Reactive Attachment Disorder. In PTSD children with physical abuse and sexual trauma, there are quite often clear signs of varying intensity attachment problems with everyone surrounding the child. This of course, makes logical sense in that a basic task of a young child is to develop trust in others. Therefore, it may take many months to gain a valid, therapeutic working connection with a stress disordered child. Foster parents relate the same kind of problem connecting with the child, and report that it may take many months to establish even a small amount of heartfelt warmth with the child.

One sign that is startling in young children who have traumatic reactions due to abuse is lack of empathy. The average child learns empathy and expressions of caring at a very early age; one only needs to watch a two-year-old with a doll or cuddle toy. Many stress disordered children show little or no empathy for others.

PTSD children may be identified by school staff as bullying other children on the playground. In one case, a boy of age eight that I treated repeatedly grabbed the hoods of other children's coats from behind, pulling and choking them, with no apparent concern or remorse, and in fact, glee. It may very well be that their own pain tolerance is so high that they cannot recognize discomfort or pain in others very well.

Or, as in the case just mentioned, the child is passing on the negative energy and rage from their perpetrator. In the case of bullying, it is well known that abuse "slides downhill". Yet in other cases, I have seen siblings who have experienced neglect and abuse together become so empathetic and protective of each other that their egos are essentially fused.

Detachment behaviors follow low empathy quite naturally. The "detachment" behaviors can range from the child having a hard time in developing social and nurturing attachments to the child being so far detached at times as to be nearing dissociation. The sudden onset of a flat affect and dilated pupils in a stress disordered child signifies deep detachment and a concurrent allostatic process. One can see how each of the symptom categories overlap and flow into each other.

Detachment reactions, which are likely signs of a chemical "dumping" process in the child's body, can make the child highly vulnerable to successive traumas and victimization. When the child is in a detached reactive state, they may not be able to invest much cognition in protecting themselves: they may simply submit to another round of abuse.

Because of their cluster of detached, socially awkward behaviors, PTSD children will often stand out in a group of other children. Teachers may note that these children seem to be targets for other children who are bullies (even other children who are not known to be bullies). The PTSD child may gravitate towards other children who victimize them by teasing or by always using them in "pickle in the middle" type of games.

These children may burn through friendships at a high rate; other children become confused by the PTSD child because one moment they are friendly and calm, the next they may be mean and highly agitated for no apparent reason. They often present a social awkwardness with peers that looks like inexperience, aggression, domination, alienation, or that they are trying far too hard to fit in. Older children with PTSD have described the feeling of being with peers as a severe "not being normal or fitting in."

Relationship Confusion

The relationships, psychological alterations, and self (ego) structure of children with acute stress or posttraumatic stress will also show notable and unique damage. For some children, when they are in contact with the adult perpetrator, they will become very affectionate and regressed. These behaviors may transfer to other adult caregivers (foster parents) following contact with the perpetrator. In other children, new relationships with adults become very difficult to establish due to the child's hypervigilance concerning trust and safety.

Some stress disordered children seem to have no fear or caution around strangers, and will approach anyone with an instant-relationship hug. These children will often become very physically clingy towards substitute caregivers, such as teachers or foster parents. It is not uncommon for them to begin to call the foster parents "mommy" and "daddy" within forty-eight hours of arrival in the foster home. It is almost as if the child is so starved for physical care and comfort that they are willing to accept this from anyone. The danger of this presentation becomes obvious.

One other interesting effect that I have noted through the years is that some abused children will transfer hostility and accusations to non-perpetrating adults such as foster parents or other caregivers quite readily. I need not elaborate for the clinical reader the phenomenon of transference, but the peculiarity of a traumatic memory situation is that the child's memory may be impaired both about the details and sequence of traumatic events. The substitute caregiver is a safe person to transfer the emotional energy of the traumatic event to.

This relationship confusion may not go as far as an accusation of abuse towards a foster parent, but it may present on a day-to-day basis in the form of the child repeatedly attempting to engage the foster parent in the same fashion that the child engaged the biological parent (or perpetrator). This pattern is one that the clinician needs to be acutely aware of if the child they are treating is in foster care, and one that the clinician needs to help the foster parent cope with through specific training on how to respond to the child's negative engagement attempts.

For young children who have experienced repeated critical incidents, the world of relationships becomes a very unsatisfying, unsafe and unpredictable place. As such, the child's behaviors may be altered in reflection of this. The child begins to create their own internal "safe place" for their ego.

I have worked in multiple cases where the child is intensely imaginative and retreats into a self-structured internal fantasy world as a means of coping. These behaviors become so marked that concerned adults may report that the child appears not only to be severely detached from others, but to be hallucinating.

One beautiful little girl named Matilda had such a fragile ego structure when she came into care, that she would retreat into a deep fantasy state and begin to use baby talk, or sing little songs completely composed of nonsense words. The behavior would often occur prior to and following court ordered visits with her biological father. To the observer, Matilda appeared to be in a near-psychotic state. This retreat into fantasy is a reasonable defense to ego destruction via the trauma. If the external world is a very unsafe place, why not retreat to a place that feels safer?

Anyone who has witnessed a child in contact with a suspected or known perpetrator of abuse may have seen the child become very affectionate, friendly, and charming with the perpetrator. The child has structured their ego expressions to protect themselves from further abuse: if they can be pleasing to the perpetrator, perhaps the perpetrator will not abuse them again. The child's ego structure is dominated by their history of abuse, and often dominated by the perpetrator of the abuse. This effect, if repeated with other people at other times, may place the child at risk for further abuse by savvy perpetrators who instinctively seem to know how to spot such a child.

Trauma and Behavior Regression: A Case Study

Each new trauma and each new stress episode places the child ever closer to catastrophic breakdown of their ego structure, or profound and permanent changes in their personality structure. Larger episodes of ego decompensation do occur during treatment, and frequently result in hospitalization. Like Matilda, children who have experienced trauma can become regressed in their behaviors when they retreat into their "safer" ego retreats. Many children I have worked with have issues with bedwetting, daytime wetting, and encopresis with feces manipulation or smearing. The following case demonstrates the connection between trauma and these kinds of behaviors.

J.T. came onto my caseload as a seven-year-old boy with mental retardation who had been age-appropriate in his toileting up until the time of his sexual abuse. J.T. lived with his mother, who was very intellectually limited and lived on the very margins of subsistence. J.T.'s mother also drank heavily at times when she became depressed. The county child protective services became involved in the case when J.T. began to push toy dinosaurs into his rectum and the mother sought help. The mother had begun to suspect that her son had been sexually abused by a male adult friend who had been babysitting the boy.

The protective services also then assessed the mother to be inadequate to care for the child. There was both neglect and physical abuse present perpetrated by the mother. Apparently, she had regularly banged the boy's head into the wall when he had misbehaved. J.T. was eventually placed in foster care, but was quickly moved from one foster home to another due to his behaviors. He eventually spent about a year in a residential treatment facility because no foster home could be found.

Following some very limited behavioral improvement, a new foster home was secured for J.T. Almost immediately, J.T. began to defecate and urinate in his bedroom, often around daybreak. He clearly had the skills to use the toilet, and could relate that he knew that the toilet was the appropriate place to put his wastes. His doctor prescribed DDAVP, but it had virtually no effect on improving the night time wetting.

Further, J.T. not only defecated in his underpants (or pull-ups), but he began to manipulate and smear the feces on the bedclothes, walls, and himself. When asked why he did this, he simply stated: "because I want to." J.T. also made repeated statements about a ghost named "George", and frequently spoke to the ghost, with accompanying glances towards the ceiling or corners of the room.

The treatment approach was based on some spotty information from J.T. that his mother had banged his head on the wall when he had toileting accidents. J.T. also indicated that the sexual perpetrator had penetrated him anally. From this information, the theory developed that J.T. was engaging in the difficult behaviors as an anger expression. It was also noted that he may be soiling and smearing in the very early morning, leading to the theory that he may be having intrusive dreams about the abuse, subsequent strong emotions, and then the behavior. Patient and detailed questioning of J.T. revealed the ghost's name was also the name of the perpetrator.

When small children have experienced abuse at the hands of an adult, they quite naturally become full of rage. Total loss of control of one's situation and body threatens one's sense of identity at a profound level. Following the traumatic event(s), could it be that the child attempts to re-claim their ego power by finding a way to "get back" or anger the perpetrator? Could the child be using the wetting and soiling to do this? Does the behavior have the added benefit of keeping a sexual perpetrator away from them? If the child speaks *to* the perpetrator when the perpetrator is not physically present, is it a hallucination, or a genuine ghost of powerful emotion?

J.T.'s foster parents were directed to wake earlier than J.T. to "catch" him before he could engage in the behaviors. They were to simply take his hand and walk to the toilet, with a non-punitive affect. When "accidents" occurred, they were to treat these as matter-of-fact, and assist J.T. in cleaning up his room and self.

Since J.T. also greatly enjoyed taking baths, bathing was used as a reward when he used the potty. Otherwise, when he urinated or soiled in his room, he was only permitted to clean up with wet wipes. Interactive work with J.T included the exploration of George the Ghost; my chasing George away from J.T., and teaching J.T. how to change the way he spoke to George the Ghost, and how to generally "stand up" to George's intimidation.

J.T. showed clear progress in these areas within a few weeks, but the progress was very slow, with frequent regressions. The foster parents eventually determined that the level of care that they needed to provide for J.T. was too draining, and he was moved to another foster home, and out of my care.

I have had many other stress disordered cases of young children who have experienced the same pattern of encopresis and enuresis (inability to control the flow of urine and involuntary urination) behaviors, as well as varieties of fantasy retreat. The children range from above average to below average intelligence, and from neglect to physical and sexual abuse. In some cases, DDAVP has some limited effect for enuresis, and psychotropic medications may help with sleep and dream intrusions. In all cases, the child had gone through potty learning and had become age appropriate at some point in their toileting. I'm convinced that the enuresis and encopresis issue, as well as the marked retreat into fantasy are important behavioral markers for stress disorders associated with abuse in children.

Traumatic Stress and Memory

When a person is experiencing a traumatic event, the whole of their energy is focused on self-preservation. The event itself may be so intense that the individual may need to "step out of themselves" in order to psychologically cope with the level of danger and stress. As such, memory is often affected. In children under the age of four, developmental issues become predominant in the area of memory. At four and under, memory is not likely to be encoded verbally, but is encoded with wordless images and sensate material.

Memory damages in children regarding their traumatic events and the time surrounding these events often includes gaps, or "missing time" as well as difficulties in being able to sequence events accurately. Any child, let alone a traumatically stressed child, will sometimes confabulate parts of a memory sequence in order to avoid embarrassment, fill in the blank for their own comfort, or in efforts to satisfy a pressing adult. This difficulty in memory sequencing seems to bleed over into everyday life for some stressed children, and this leads to further complications when adults in their life begin to accuse them of lies and confabulations.

If a child was under the age of four when their abuse occurred, they will likely not be able to relate much significant material in treatment. They will also not be able to articulate very well what they are experiencing in the stress episode, or the source of their stress. They of course have the memories, but these memories are largely sensory experiences.

For example, from the time I was a small boy, I had a terrifying re-occurring dream that continued into adulthood and mystified me. I would awake with an intense physical sensation that my mouth was overfull, tongue swelled, and lips full and heavy. On the surface, this does not seem so terrifying, but it certainly was to me. As a clinician, I knew there had to be some explanation for this, but through my own self-examination, study, and even brief therapy, I could not discover it.

It was only about a year ago (at age 46) that I discovered the answer to my bad dream. In conversation with my mother, who was dying of emphysema, she (re) told me the story of my first weeks of life. I had been born on time, but was premature weight. Due to this, I was placed in an incubator for several weeks.

When my parents came to visit me, they were shocked to see that the inside of my mouth was painted a bright blue color. The hospital staff revealed to my parents that the nipples that the hospital had been using to feed the babies had been defective; they had only one very small hole in them. The nurses apparently thought that because I was so small, I was not eating very much. In fact, I was sucking so hard on the nipple, (and not getting enough food) my mouth became very sore (thus the bright blue medication swabbed in my mouth).

Though my mother had related this story to me before, it had never connected for me with my dream. But this re-telling impacted upon me like a bombshell. There no longer was any doubt for me what my dream was about. Why did it take me so long to connect the story, which I have known since I was a small boy, with the bad dream? While I do not know the answer to this deep (perhaps Freudian) mystery, I have a feeling it had something to do with my mother's impending death. Since this discovery, I have not had the dream.

At the risk of being obvious to the reader, traumatic memory does not have to be articulated verbally, it is often (perhaps more significantly) recalled through the senses. Traumatic memory, while vivid and powerful, is rarely full and robust; it is fragmented and strongly entwining discrete details with intense and terrifying emotion. Children have unique behavioral signs and symptoms of PTSD that adults do not. If the clinician, not to mention the entire treatment field, never ventures beyond the current DSM definitions and understandings of stress disorders in children, the children will not receive the quality of treatment that they deserve.

Confusing Stress Behaviors with Common Childhood Behaviors

Often, children with Acute Stress Disorder or Post Traumatic Stress Disorder have one or more diagnoses behind them before they are accurately diagnosed with a stress disorder. Caregivers and clinicians see the behavioral signs that the child is demonstrating and come to the conclusion that the child may be ADHD, very oppositional, bi-polar, or simply under-disciplined. Though many of the behavioral signs of stress disorders are common to other disorders, when the total inventory of signs are viewed, along with any known traumatic or stressful history, the diagnosis becomes quite evident. It is also good to remember that the differences are seen in the quality, intensity, frequency, duration, as well as known history of a trauma.

In cases where the child is living with their biological parent(s), and there is an intergenerational history of domestic abuse, addiction, or child abuse, the adults may either be in denial of the possibility of a stress disorder (or an event that has caused it), or they have become numb themselves and do not have the perspective needed to recognize the behaviors in the child as abnormal. In these cases, children are often first identified as having some kind of problem in pre-school or kinder-garten.

It is amazing to me how the child is sometimes the only one who "knows" what their diagnosis is, and how adults around them (often highly educated adults) cannot figure it out. Adults, even professionals in mental health, will often not be able to "connect the dots" between demonstrated behaviors and the known history of the child's traumas. I tend to believe that many adults who work with children are so uncomfortable with the facts surrounding childhood trauma, that they uncon-sciously (or consciously) avoid addressing the realities of it. To be sure, it is much more comfortable to treat a child's agitated behaviors as some other diagnosis than to listen to the child describe his or her sexual abuse. Below is an overview of how each of the six behavioral sign clusters may be confused with normal childhood behaviors.

Allostatic Behavioral Signs

These behavioral signs at first may be mistaken for hyperactivity or simple childhood excitement, but these signs tend to be much more intense, and not in relation to the situation around the child. The child at times seems to become very agitated, anxious, aggressive, overly shy, or very fearful for no real or apparent reason, or there appears to be an overreaction to some event or situation. This may be passed off as a sensitive or highly strung child.

The child may become very silly or overly familiar with strangers. This can be misinterpreted as the child being a "clown" or a "flirt". These children often have a very hard time calming down. There may be problems with sleep: getting to sleep, staying asleep, and nightmares. The child may startle very easily, and may be overly clingy towards caregivers. The adults in their life may label them as excitable, simply full of extra energy, or a "dynamo".

The child's appetite and bowel-bladder habits may be affected. There is often an increase in toileting accidents, intentional toileting in closets, corners, etc. The child may actually manipulate or play with their own or animal feces. There may be regressions, slow, or stalled potty learning in younger children. The adults in the child's life may label this as the child not wanting to grow up, wanting to remain a "Mamma's boy", or equate these behaviors with the child being "willful" or being "hard to break". (There may be, in fact, some truth to this, as the child may be demonstrating rage at their abuse and abuser).

Children may also express a sudden change of affect: their expression may become flat, pupils may dilate, and the child will look as if they are daydreaming, or "off in their own world". These children may be described by their parents as being a "daydreamer". Some other children may have sudden bursts of energy that look like they just had a dose of "speed", becoming very physically active and agitated very quickly. The behaviors may be passed off as simple childhood imitation of characters on TV, or a child who is "always looking for trouble".

These behavioral signs can occur at any time the child is "triggered" by someone, some thing, or some location in their environment. The number and kind of triggers can be difficult to ascertain, especially in younger children. Parents may have some insight into the fact that certain activities seem to get their child wound up, but cannot identify why this is so, or misidentify the reason. For example, a parent may state that his child always gets out of control when there is a visit between the child and particular cousins; in fact, it might be the perpetrating uncle of the child that is triggering the reaction. When there is a dramatic increase in agitation following contact with a person who is a trigger, this is often confused with the child being upset, sad, or disappointed that they are no longer in the person's presence or care. The key differences between a triggered PTSD episode and the child simply missing the person is that the signs are much more intense, of longer duration, and include hours if not days of severe and consistent misbehavior as well as an increase of the other five sign clusters.

Re-experiencing

These behavioral signs may be confused with a child's normal play; children may engage in violent play, sexualized play, or other re-enactments of traumatic events in their lives with action figures or dolls. This type of play may be discounted as normal due to exposure to television or friends who are a bad influence.

The child may become oppositional over small issues; they may seem to need to be in control of every situation to feel comfortable. This may be confused with being bossy, stubbornness and "being contrary". The difference is that when an average child is pressed to comply, they will give in; when a stressed child is pressed, their agitation increases to the point of getting out of control.

Children who have been sexually abused may engage in more frequent and public masturbation or simulated sex acts. They may also engage in odd behaviors, such as stuffing toilet paper or other objects in their pants. They may use explicitly sexual language, or have precocious knowledge about sex.

These behaviors are much more difficult to pass off as something else. In some cases, I have heard parents explain these behaviors as the child, once again, acting like an adult that they have seen on television, or exposure to the poor influences of the child's friends. There may be an attempt to normalize the behaviors: "all children touch themselves there", or "they are playing doctor".

Nightmares are a form of re-experiencing, but they are also quite a normal event in any child's life. The difference for stress-disordered children is the intensity and frequency of the intrusive dreams, which may be accompanied by wetting or soiling, or an inability to go back to sleep and urges to play following the dream.

Avoidance, Numbing and Detachment

This behavioral cluster can be confused with a child trying to avoid responsibilities, being stubborn, being a loner, or angry with family members. The child may actively avoid certain people, places, or items. They may seem to have forgotten all about the traumatic event that took place, or their recent acting out/stress episode. Adults can pass this off as the child having forgotten all about the traumatic event, and "being over it".

The child may not respond to every day injuries like other children; they may easily shake off scrapes and bumps without tears or any reaction at all. This is passed off as the child being "one tough little kid". On the other hand, they may become very upset and over reactive to very slight injuries, the child then being labeled "a sissy".

The child may seem to bully other children by simply ignoring the other child and "plowing on through". The child may actually physically attack another child with pinching, biting, hitting, or strangling. This may be confused with sibling rivalry or peer disagreements, but the marker is the frequency and intensity of the behaviors. They may seem to have little empathy for other people who are injured or have their feelings hurt.

In most stress-disordered children, there is often a lack of the ability to self-comfort. In play, it can also be seen that the child has not formed much attachment to any one toy; the child may not have a cuddle toy, for example. Again, this may earn the child a label of being "tough", or being a leader, or having promise for a career in professional wrestling.

Psychological Alterations

These behavioral signs may be confused with a child who is "spoiled". The child may continue to try to sleep in the caregiver's bed, they may show regressed developmental behaviors, such as daytime wetting, using "baby talk", or a desire to use a pacifier or bottle, or becoming very clingy to the caregiver. The child may exhibit memory problems or confabulate wild stories or fantasies that are considerably more detailed or odd than the average child's "active imagination".

The child may become hypervigilant; they may be very watchful and seem anxious, or fearful of being abandoned. Parents of these children will often either ridicule the child for their regressed behaviors, or indulge the behaviors, keeping the child "their baby" or protecting them as extraordinarily fragile. The child and their parents may demonstrate odd or altered views of the world and society that they proudly legitimize as "being different" than other people, or being a "born rebel". There may be a kind of fatalism and resignation presented by the child and family.

The child may be very impulsive, and engage in risky play without apparent understanding of the danger. The child may either have gained a very hostile and negative attitude towards the world, or they present themselves to others as very vulnerable, and then get taken advantage of or are re-victimized. The adults in the child's life may call them a "daredevil", or in the latter case, support them vehemently as victims of a hostile world (teachers, counselors, and police).

Relational Problems

This set of behavioral signs may be confused with an over shyness, or a child who "has not had the right discipline", or is "full of themselves". The child may have trouble trusting others, may be secretive and very guarded. The child may have problems making and keeping friends.

They may "try too hard" to be friendly or to fit in. The child may become very bossy and parentified. There may physical boundary problems in the way the child relates to others, such as standing too close, touching too freely or too soon in a relationship. The child may touch others inappropriately, such as tickling or sexualized touching. The child may seem to crave help, care, and affection, but when it is given, push the helper away.

These children will often be quickly identified as behavior problems when they start school. Quite often, the family is so used to these aberrations, and other family members exhibit similar behaviors, making them normalized in the family.

Ego Structure

These behavioral signs may be confused with a child who is simply "down" or depressed. The child may seem to be very emotionally fragile and "fall apart" easily. Again, this may be passed off as a "sensitive child". They may verbalize low self - esteem, or blame themselves for the bad things that have happened to them.

The parents may identify and defend their child as a victim of other children's (or teachers, counselors, etc.) hostility. The child may alternate from being very opposi-tional and defensive to being excessively cooperative and easily led. The adults surrounding the child may explain this as the child being "a fighter", or alternately, a child who "just wants to make friends."

There may be periods of time where the child retreats into extraordinarily detailed fantasy. They may even have their own secret language have different names for themselves. While other children and adults may find this to be odd, the parents of the child may find this "charming" and marvel at the child's "wild imagination" or be amused at their "imaginary friend".

Essentially, the markers for a child with a stress disorder as opposed to normal childhood behaviors becomes: known critical incidents, the presence of all six clusters of behavioral signs, the intensity of the signs above average childhood behaviors, and the duration, and frequency at which they occur.

5 | Anatomy of the Stress Episode

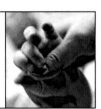

As therapists, one of our major tools is our words. Most adults, when they witness a child who is severely upset over what appears to be resistance to a directive, will label the behavior a "tantrum", or at best "acting out". In most cases, this is a fairly accurate term for the behavior that the child is exhibiting.

When a stress-disordered child engages in similar behaviors, the source and *quality* of the behaviors will be different at different times. A stress-disordered child may indeed have a tantrum or act out from time to time, but they also have a different, discrete behavior set expressing their PTSD. The more accurate and effective term for these discrete behaviors is "stress episode".

The word "tantrum" implies that the child has control over their behavior, and that the behavior is intended to make some advantage or gain for the child. Tantrums are behavior manipulations by the child that usually only last a few minutes. Though stress episodes can be very brief (minutes), the difference between stress episodes and simple tantrums will be quite evident if the observer is careful in their observations. The telling difference between a "tantrum" and a "stress episode" is the quality, duration, intensity, frequency, and known history of trauma.

By insisting on precision in describing the upset behavior, we help the child by educating other helping adults. By consistently using the more accurate "stress episode", we help others to fully understand the *source* of the behavior being seen is not simple opposition, stubbornness, manipulation, or a spoiled child. When this is accomplished, we are on the way to help teachers, parents, foster parents, and other caregivers to depersonalize the child's reactive behaviors. After all, the child may be directing their behavior towards me, but they are really reacting to something or someone in their past.

Phase I: Cue and Trigger

Children's stress episodes seem to follow a roughly four-phase process. The first phase begins with a cue and trigger. A cue or trigger to a stress disordered person is some internal or external reminder of their trauma. There can be literally hundreds of possible cue-triggers.

Some the victim may be aware of, while others cannot be cited with any accuracy. The younger the victim, the more invisible to the observer triggers tend to be. Sometimes, caregivers can determine specific triggers, or very close observations by a Behavior Specialist may be needed. When the triggers are discovered, they should be shared with the entire treatment team and carefully recorded.

In younger children, who cannot verbally relate their trauma in treatment, identification of cues and triggers can help the clinician gain a generalized view of and hypothesis of what the details of the trauma may have been. This information is not to be used to test the child's memory, or to lead the child to some conclusion, but rather to help the clinician more fully understand the reactivity protocol that the child has. In turn, this helps to focus treatment and eventual work on inoculating the child to those particular cue-triggers.

Triggers can be sights, sounds, smells, tactile sensations, places, times of the day or year, or even intrusive memories and dreams. Thus, the world around the child becomes full of potential conscious and unconscious reminders: books, songs, stories, a piece of clothing, a color of paint in a room, the smell of bacon, a vocal tone... on and on it goes.

It should be noted that just because a child experiences a cue, it doesn't mean that they will trigger. The process of the cue triggering a reaction is likely dependent upon the child's overall level of stress. If you think of a glass, almost filled with water, there is no problem until the glass gets overfilled. Thus, it can become confusing for the clinician observing the child's behaviors: a cue on one day may trigger a stress episode, but not trigger on another day.

Once the cue is received, and the stress reaction is triggered, the child will escalate with physical and emotional agitation. Essentially, the child's fear reaction motivates a flight or fight reaction, often with lightening speed. Chemicals of various sorts rush into the child's bloodstream, and the allostatic process begins, uncontrolled. Heartbeat, respiration, and blood pressure rise. Muscles tense, vision may blur and the child may become unresponsive to directives or support.

The escalation timetable may vary from child-to-child or from episode-to-episode, but most children follow a predictable, unique pattern. Once the escalation reaches certain, hard to determine point, the stress episode is almost impossible to stop. Like a runaway freight train, it will continue until the tracks run out.

It is important to understand that the increasing physical agitation at first may be undetectable to the observer. In some children, there is a "slow burn" kind of reactivity, while in others; the reaction is very explosive and instantaneous. "Slow burn" type children make the job of trying to discern cues and triggers that much more difficult for the clinician, as the first signs of a stress episode may be several minutes to hours after the cue-trigger.

Phase II: Escalation

The Escalation Phase may include age regressed behaviors, physical combativeness, foul or nonsensical language, flight (running away long or short distances) or hiding behaviors, oppositional expressions, flat affect, pupil dilation, radical personality change, wetting or soiling, and self-harm attempts. The behaviors may reach a plateau and continue for a brief or moderately long period of time.

Fight behaviors include physical combativeness in various degrees, from aggressive, targeted attacks of individuals to a generalized physical posturing of threat. There may be present physical gestures of warding off, or defensive behaviors such as waving of the arms, covering the face, or curing up in the fetal position with occasional kicks. These often present in stark opposition to the situation at hand. In one event in my work, a simple placement of my hand on a young boy's shoulder triggered him into a highly defensive posture, waving his hands in front of his face, as if to ward off blows to his face.

Some children may exhibit strong flight behavior during their escalation phase. Flight behaviors can take many forms: while treating a child once in a school, he ran away from me, out of the building, and all the way to his home, several blocks away. In another situation, a child consistently ran a short distance from the treatment area to a coat-room, hiding among the coats.

During a session in a foster home, I watched a little four year old boy move rapidly from frozen fear to falling asleep, standing up, while the foster parent was gently trying to correct his behavior. If I had not been there to see it, I don't think I would have believed it. All of these behaviors qualify as flight.

Secondary sets of behaviors, closely related to "fight" behaviors are those of self-harm or disregard for personal safety during an episode. Some children will bite themselves, bang their heads, or throw themselves to the floor or into walls with apparently no discomfort or caution. The child, unable to strike out at the perpetrator, takes the rage out by fighting him or herself. This behavior also likely has to do with the tendency for numbing during both the original trauma and during stress episodes. A friend of mine, who is a victim of trauma, says: "the soldier does not pay too much attention to his wounds until he is out of the battle."

In some cases, a child may cycle through this phase multiple times before moving on to the next phase. It often appears that the escalation process itself is a trigger for repeated escalation. In effect, the chemical "switch" that has been turned on gets stuck, producing round after round of episodes. This "training" or chaining effect can last hours, even days in some severe cases.

Phase III: Emotional Release

The third noted phase I call Emotional Release. During this time, a child may move from hostile, defensive behaviors to a deeper age regression that may include wetting or soiling him or herself, sucking their thumb, baby talk, and tears or deep weeping. The child could begin at this time to spontaneously relate traumatic memories.

It should be noted that the child may not be willing to share history at this time, and sharing should not be pushed upon the child. The movement from phase to phase is usually not clear and concise. Some children will move clearly rapidly from hostile and aggressive to vulnerable and needy. In most cases, though, there will be gradual transition from the highly agitated state to a more withdrawn, and regressed expression.

Phase IV: Exhaustion/Return

The fourth phase of the stress episode might be called Exhaustion/Return. Following the intensity of the tears or weeping, the child seems to return to normal, often very rapidly. It almost may seem like an invisible switch has been thrown: the child suddenly has a normal affect, may even be cheerful, and behaves as if nothing has even happened.

A second possible behavioral effect is that the child will become quite sleepy, and appear completely exhausted. Often, if you quiz the child at this time about what it was that upset them so, they will not be able to tell you. They are not lying; they often actually do not recall the trigger.

This may be due to the fact that a very similar dissociative process takes place during the stress episode as it did during the actual critical incident. When an individual is in a highly stressed state, they are not able to mentally record details, because they have other concerns: self-preservation. While in this dream like state, the child's memories are severely skewed.

The child's vulnerability to triggers and stress episodes has two important variables: how strong the child's ego wrapping is in any particular moment, and what the level of their overall stress load is. Remember that the stress "glass" can only hold so much water. Once too much water is added, the overflow of stress signs occurs. Recognition, monitoring, and management of the child's stress loads, capacity, and ego state become one key to treatment.

Case Studies

Ralph, age five, had been under my care for some twenty-two months. Ralph and his sister Matilda, age six, had come from a very abusive family situation. Their biological mother was very low functioning, was addicted, and had been in prison for prostitution. They had been routinely locked in a bedroom with a box of crackers and a bottle of water for hours on end. They had lived with their biological father and his mother for some time before coming into foster care. It was determined that both the father and grandmother had also physically abused the children, and sexual abuse by the father on Matilda was suspected.

Both children were highly reactive when they came into foster care. They triggered so often and the stress episodes were so intense, that it was difficult to discern discrete episodes or triggers. It seemed as if the children were always either on their way through a dramatic escalation, having an emotional release, or were exhausted from the entire process. Each of them could easily trigger each other. Through close observation over a long period of time, each child's unique set of triggers and process started to be discerned.

Over the course of treatment, both children's stress episodes decreased in length and intensity, but did still continue. One notable fact is that even over the course of the twenty-two months of treatment, ever new stress behaviors and triggers were presented. For example, Ralph accompanied his foster family to a visit to family friends. The foster father noticed that he had not seen Ralph for some few minutes, and went looking for him. The foster father found Ralph in the bathroom, standing in front of the toilet, with head, shoulders, and shirt wet. In addition, Ralph held a flat affect and had glazed eyes. It became clear that Ralph had stood in front of the toilet, and had dunked his head in the bowl.

Though Ralph had never done this behavior before in the foster home, he had in the past had very stressed behaviors while in bathrooms to bathe, or to clean up after toileting accidents. It was reasonable, in this case, to conclude that the behavior was stress reactive to some trigger Ralph had just experienced. One could also extrapolate that the behavior perhaps was a re-enactment of an abusive punishment in his past.

Wally, age eight, had been repeatedly pushed into a closet by his intoxicated father when he became angry with Wally. During one of these critical incidents, the father got a box of screws and a power screwdriver, and screwed the door shut on Wally. When his mother discovered him hours later, he had nearly pulled all of his fingernails off trying to pry and scratch his way out of the closet. In school, Wally was having difficulty in a particular classroom. He repeatedly shut down and was placed by the teacher sitting on the floor outside of the classroom.

During these times he became uncommunicative, held himself tightly, cried, and rocked back and forth, and at times clawed at the air around him. This behavior could last hours. In observing the teacher and Wally interact, it became clear that the way she corrected Wally was a trigger for his shutting down: she used a forceful, loud tone of voice when she thought Wally was becoming resistive to her directives.

The more he became "oppositional", the more the teacher raised and firmed her voice. In turn, Wally became even more defensive. At some point, the intensity of the teacher's voice and pressure would trigger Wally's stress reactivity, and his body simply did what it had done during his abuse. Eventually, Wally would "come out of" his stress episode, and returned to class as if nothing had happened. The entire process would then repeat when the teacher once again perceived Wally as becoming oppositional.

A child's stress episode is packed with behavioral information that can help in so many ways. It can help define a particular behavior set in connection with a particular incident. It can present a well defined enactment that can be used as material in treatment. It can help the clinician help others to depersonalize the child's behaviors towards them. Lastly, it can provide a route to giving gentle empathy to the child. Those who dismiss the stress episode as simply a set of difficult behaviors to extinguish are missing out on a great therapeutic tool for healing.

6 A Course of Treatment for Abused Children with PTSD

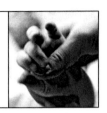

The very good news for abused children who suffer from Post Traumatic Stress Disorder is that their symptoms can improve to a great degree. It is important for all those who care for these children to understand the course of treatment, because this understanding can help the child to progress and to avoid frustration.

Often, adults want the child's symptoms to be reduced quickly. This is not only for the child's sake, but because when a child has severe symptoms, it can be overwhelming and stressful for caregivers, teachers, and even therapists. In treating PTSD in children, the progress of the treatment cannot be rushed. When it is rushed, the child usually "shuts down", and the treatment may be delayed for some time. It is good to remember that the child must always be in charge of the pace of treatment.

Gentling makes strong use of cognitive restructuring and specific adult behaviors in working with the child. Efforts are made throughout treatment to help the child to think differently about themselves, their ability to deal with the world, their stress reactivity, and their relationship to their trauma. The adults who work with the child must adopt a behavioral strategy that pairs high structure with high nurturing.

The adult approach is both firm and kind. Age appropriate expectations are made and gentle responses to stress issues are demonstrated. Boundaries are stated, kept, and often repeated. Compassion and kindness are demonstrated not only during the child's stress episodes, but also when the child is being corrected or reminded of boundaries in the course of a normal day.

My course of treatment has four parts that will overlap a great deal.

Part I: Safety

The first stage of treatment is for the child to feel completely safe in all environments. This means "all environments": a child may feel comfortable and safe in their classroom, but not yet safe outdoors at recess, or in the school rest rooms, or in the cafeteria. Helping the child to feel safe everywhere may take some length of time, depending on the nature, intensity, frequency, and duration of their trauma history. Keep in mind that we are talking at least months, and more likely years.

Part II: Self-Realizing

The second line of progress is for the child to begin to self realize their symptoms and level of stress. In many cases, the child has lived for so long with very high levels of stress; they do not even realize how much stress they carry. The work to help the child become self-aware of their symptom processes, again, may take varying amounts of time depending on the child's age, their ability to feel safe in most environments, and what their trauma was.

Part III: Psycho-Education

The midway point in treatment begins the process of education. The child needs to begin to learn specific techniques to help themselves to cope with the stress reaction that they now are aware of. The child needs to learn ways to access adult help in coping. This education not only includes the child, but all of the adults who work with the child, such as teachers, family, and therapeutic staff.

Part IV: Stress Inoculation

The last stage of treatment focuses on stress inoculation. This is a process of sensitively and gradually supporting the child through exposure to known stressful situations and triggers. Again, this process may take many months and even years to accomplish. *A major key to progress in treatment is that all of the adults in the child's life must gain adequate understanding of the disorder and how to approach the child.*

When a child encounters an adult who does not "get it", at best stress episodes increase, and at worse, treatment grinds to a halt. In most cases, the four parts of treatment overlap a great deal. The previous stage work is not abandoned when the next is introduced, and the next stages of work are often begun when the child indicates readiness for them.

Treatment Objectives

For most clinicians, articulating the objectives of treatment is a required part of treatment preparation for their formal, written treatment plan. The following ten objectives of treatment are by no means exhaustive; each child will have a unique presentation of needs. This is especially true if the child has a co-morbid mental health disorder.

1. Lower physical and psychological agitation and reactivity

Children with Acute Stress or Post Traumatic Stress usually have a good bit of difficulty in school both academically and socially. The agitation and reactivity that they suffer from is very disruptive to the everyday tasks that children need to do in the home, community, and school. Even though an observer may not notice it, stress disordered children always have a low burning "pilot light" of physical and psychological agitation.

This flame, though small, is constantly distracting and draining to the child's normal development. In treatment, the child is initially unable to effect a reduction of the agitation and reactivity on their own. They need help from adult caregivers who are taught specific techniques. The primary, daily treatment to combat this is to provide the child with very gentle, very measured high structure and nurturing.

That tiny "pilot light" of agitation can easily explode into a bright flame of reactivity, both psychological and physical, usually first seriously noted when the child begins school. These reactivations can be genuinely disturbing and frightening for adult caregivers who do not fully understand the history of the child or how to manage the resulting behaviors of stress reactions. The child will quickly be labeled in some way, adding yet another stress burden.

Since the child's reactivity behaviors are the most apparent issue, the behaviors will often be initially described by well meaning teachers as "ADHD", "oppositional", or the ever-trendy "bi-polar". Thus the child enters into the realm of the school psychologist, already labeled (incorrectly).

The reader will note that this initial treatment objective really has four parts: lowering psychological agitation, lowering psychological reactivity, lowering physical agitation, and lowering physical reactivity. Each of these four discrete areas of treatment, while integrated into the whole, usually needs specific, focused attention to affect overall progress.

This treatment objective is not just listed first because the behavioral signs are so disturbing to adults, or that repeated stress episodes gain the child a heavy label. I am convinced that each additional stress episode that a child suffers brings the child closer to the development of ancillary mental health problems or conversion of the primary stress disorder into a more permanent and less treatable condition. Each stress episode drives the reactivity process deeper, and thus makes it more difficult to end.

In fact, an apparent inability for the body to come back to a normal homeostasis can be seen in children who have suffered for years from a poorly or untreated stress disorder. And so this objective is not only important for the here-and-now problem of helping the child to calm down enough to function in school, but also to halt the progress of this difficult aspect of PTSD.

2. Self-initiation of learned stress reduction

The traumatized child needs to discover, be taught, and self-initiate ways to reduce their own stress. While the external high structure and high nurture by adult caregivers assists the child in daily coping and development, they will need to learn how to do these same things for themselves as part of their growing up. After all, the child may find themselves in situations where they have only themselves to rely upon for stress management. The need to learn such self care is not so very different from any child's development, but it is more focused, intentional, and specific in its teaching and development.

If the clinician is able to complete a detailed history, they may find that children who have PTSD experienced long term neglect, physical, sexual, emotional, or domestic abuse. I believe that the diagnostic field and the treatment field have some distance to travel to adequately describe and treat this type of "life dysfunction stress".

3. Resuming and continuing here-and-now development

One of the more obvious signs in the behavior of children with stress disorders is that they appear to be quite immature. In fact, the normal development of the child in all spheres has been severely disrupted by their critical incident(s). Often, treatment for children with mental health disorders is so much focused on ending the signs and symptoms that one forgets to make use of normative development as a tool for treatment. It becomes socially and academically important for the child to quickly curtail stress signs, especially in the school environment. Emphasis only on the child's difficult behaviors, and not building on normal development, can be a trap that only makes behaviors worse.

The stressed child should be given kind, firm, mild to moderate pressure to "rise" to their normative age level though practice of age normative skills. This does, admittedly, add to their stress burden. By applying age normative stressors in the context of high structure and high support, there is a positive pay off for the stress. A specific goal in the child's treatment plan should be designed to support this objective. Good additions to the objective might include sustained positive peer interactions, adequate grades, and insistence that the child actively participate in at least one (not more than two) organized peer activities (such as a sport, church group, etc.) during treatment. Work will likely need to be done as well with the adult caregivers of the child.

While the child's need for nurturing and fulfilling the missing developmental material is essential, so is the need to help the child to behave in a more age normative fashion in the here and now. Most adults, knowing the details of a trauma that a child has been through, will tend to permit far too much behavioral regression, provide an unhealthy level of indulgence, and allow the child to "work" this sympathetic response. This only creates an added level of behavioral challenge that is best avoided if possible.

While we want the adults in the child's life to be compassionate and understanding, we also want them to continue to have age normative expectations of them. By helping the child to continue normal development at the same time we are addressing the genuine "bottomless pit" of nurturing, we are increasing ego integrity and ego strength, and this is a very positive tool in helping the child to overcome the negative effects of their trauma.

1. Achieve safety

Not to insult the reader's intelligence, but fear (real fear, not rollercoaster fear) is very uncomfortable, even painful. Intense fear, either brief or extended, plays havoc with an individual's conceptualization of the world, and, their own identity. The essential question becomes: who am I if at any time, something or someone can enter into my life (or, my body) and so overwhelmingly take over and control my emotions, thoughts, and even if I live or die?

Research has shown that recovery from Acute Stress is quicker and easier when the trauma a person experiences is a natural disaster than if the trauma was perpetrated by another human being. This makes sense from a cuing perspective, as tornados, floods, and hurricanes (or even high winds) do not present themselves to us every day. Other people do present themselves to us every day. If you are a child, and your trauma was perpetrated upon you by an adult, every adult you meet is a potential cue, if not another perpetrator.

Expressions of fear for a stressed child may be either demonstrations of anxiety or even aggression, both of which become very debilitating in everyday life. It's very hard to complete your math seatwork at school if you cannot stop being hyper-vigilant, looking over your shoulder every few moments to check to see if someone is behind you, ready to cuff your ears. Once again, gentleness, high structure, and high nurture in the environment are key to helping to meet this objective.

2. Experience positive re-engagement

The real fact is that not many people in the "real world" (sadly, even mental health professionals) come to an adequate understanding of PTSD in children. A child who suffers from a stress disorder has been through thousands of cycles of reactivity that not only includes their own stress reactions, but other's reactions the child's stress episode. When a child has a stress episode, chances are that the parent, teacher, police officer, or friend does not have a clue as to why the child has suddenly become behaviorally aggressive, hostile, oppositional, or full of rage.

It is human nature to meet such emotions and behaviors (from the stressed child) with matched aggression, anger, pressure, and even physical restraint. All of which, of course, only serve to make the stress episode worse. Adult caregivers who are able to consistently engage the stressed child in a gentle, firm, and positive manner are helping to heal the child.

In traumas that are perpetrated by an adult on a child, positive re-engagement is a tough challenge. Most clinicians expect to develop "joining" or "therapeutic alliance" with a child within a few sessions. Don't kid yourself that this will work with a stress disordered child.

Trust develops at their pace, and this is not likely to occur for two to six months, if not longer. If you push this process, the child will "fire" you. You may be able to superficially work with some of their behaviors, but progress will be slow, or disappear as soon as any slack is given in pressure for behavioral compliance. If you give them time, and are gentle, they will, in time, positively engage with you, letting you know it's time to move forward.

3.   Re-connect and feel trust with others.

Beyond positive re-engagement is a deeper experience of connection and trust. Traumatic incidents that have involved the betrayal of trust severely damage a child's ability to be open enough to the kinds of intimacy that are not only pleasurable, but help them to grow and develop. As mentioned earlier, many children with Acute Stress. or PTSD also have a "rule out" diagnosis of Reactive Attachment Disorder (RAD)

RAD-like signs must be aggressively addressed in treatment to help the child "get back on track" in their significant and formative attachments with others. Some children who come from intergenerational chaotic families may not have much of a clue what healthy intimacy is. Other children who have had fairly average development up to their trauma may be extremely cautious of getting close to anyone for quite some time.

4.   Approach the history of the critical incident

Since wounds and scars hurt and ache, it is human nature to want to avoid poking at them. Although you may have a preference on how your band-aid is taken off, (ripped off fast or slowly peeled away), you surely desire to be prepared before the event. While processing the history of the child's trauma is an important objective, it should not be at the expense of the child's readiness to do so.

An approach that has at its heart 'gentleness' will earn the respect, and thus the telling of the traumatic story. Once again, the clinician needs to resist the urge to quickly get details of the story, or "to get the story out". Some children may be able to tolerate this, but most are in a fragile ego state that may not be able to avoid decompensation if such "flooding" techniques are employed.

5.   Work through the critical incident(s)

Everyone wants to be known, and to have their story heard. When we tell our story, and feel as though others are not only interested, but can empathize with our experience, this is a powerful healing process. At its most basic, it's what therapy is all about. Helping the child to connect current emotions and behaviors to their trauma (when applicable) is a large part of "working through". Helping them to cognitively restructure their understanding and memories of the incident, and make accurate appropriations of responsibility is equally important

6.   Ego wrap and help the child differentiate

Children who have lived abusive and neglected lives often have very poor self-esteem and identities. They have quite a bit of damage to their ego and are limited in their ability to differentiate. In cases of neglect, physical, emotional, and sexual abuse that have been ongoing for some time, children, just like adults, become enmeshed and fused with their perpetrators. The child becomes chronically over-whelmed by the chaos and multiple traumas in their life.

A major behavioral sign for these children is that they seem to have very poor physical boundaries: they may hit other children and adults with little restraint or provocation, they may be overly physically affectionate, or be intrusive to conversation or other children's play. Some children with very poor ego wrapping may be perpetual victims to other children, and cannot seem to put up any defense to more aggressive, bullying, or opportunistic peers.

Essentially, the child is unable to "differentiate" between their "home world" and the "world outside". They are so used to being fused with those around them; they easily become intrusive to others outside of their "abuse circle". Their poor ego wrapping results in their being hyper-reactive to any negative emotion or excitement that is found in their school or community.

The great Murray Bowen, of course, coined the term "differentiation" to describe the process of healthy ego development and strengthening. Marriage and Sex Therapist David Schnarch's definition of differentiation is: "the ability to hold on to yourself while in intimate contact with another." Schnarch speaks about a person's ability to not be overwhelmed by other people's (especially those close to us) emotions; the ability to continue to know who you are in the face of the other person's pressure on you to comply with their way. When a child has experienced interpersonal trauma, such as abuse, their personal identity is stolen from them: they become a possession of the perpetrator.

The hallmark of enmeshment is that the individuals have countless cycles of emotional (and physical) reactivity towards each other. As in the very first treatment objective, lowering and eventually ending such intense and debilitating reactivity is a basic key to treatment. Helping a child to gain healthy differentiation will allow them to "hold on to themselves" when recalling their critical events.

Differentiation will help the child "cut the ties" that bind them to their trauma and perpetrator. When we help a child to gain ego strength and enable them to experience differentiation, we not only are treating them in the here and now, but we are helping them to avoid becoming victims of interpersonal trauma in the future.

7.   Get all caregivers "on board".

This treatment objective is perhaps the most difficult (and annoying) to accomplish. Like passengers on the Titanic who could not believe "that little bump" is going to cause the ship to sink, many adults have a very difficult time accepting that the observed behaviors are caused by an event in the past, and not the child's "bucking them" just to be oppositional or passive aggressive toward them. Indeed, the techniques of Gentling, when not accepted through the perspective of the child's historical trauma(s) seem to make no sense at all. All adult caregivers must accept not only the Gentling objectives, techniques and approach, but the underlying connection between the child's behaviors and the history that produces them.

Gentling and emotive regulation

Traumas, by definition, are highly emotional events. They can be compared rightly to grief. In fact, you might say that the victim of interpersonal trauma has experienced the death of who they used to be before the trauma occurred. Just as emotionally overwhelming is a part of grief when a loved one dies, so too are the overwhelming emotions following interpersonal trauma. Just as grieving for a loved one may last many years, so does the grieving for the self, following interpersonal trauma.

If a person is not the direct recipient of grief, as when perhaps a close friend's parent dies in old age to natural causes, we might visit the funeral parlor in support of the friend. While we are saddened, we are not in deep grief like our friend is. A simple visit to the funeral parlor enables us to limit the amount of exposure to our friend's (and others present) grief.

If the "viewing" is relatively sedate and emotionally constrained, so much the better, because we may feel quite uncomfortable if the loved ones of the deceased are *wailing* in their pain. Once again, we point to human nature: we become very disconcerted when someone around us is expressing intense negative emotion that we are not feeling ourselves. Though one could argue that the reason one person feels uncomfortable in a *wailing* situation is that they are experiencing a different cultural expression of grief, there remains many people who cannot tolerate attending *any* funeral viewings, even ones in their own culture. Empathy has its comfort limits, and the culture places fairly strict time limits on grieving.

There are, of course, qualitative differences between the grief behaviors following a (non-traumatic) death of a loved one and the grief behaviors of a child following their rape. These qualitative differences in behaviors are that eventually, the person grieving the death of a loved one passes *through* the anger of loss. Victims of interpersonal trauma clearly have a bigger uphill climb with the resulting anger and rage.

Since they have a bigger battle to wage, clinicians need to accept that child trauma victims will heal much slower than our societal norms have tolerance for. Clinicians need to be advocates to the society at large to increase tolerance for the extended time it takes for a child to recover. This is no small task with fellow professionals, let alone "managed care" gatekeepers!

Emotions, of course, have their source inside the individual, and usually have behaviors attached. People might be divided into three basic categories when it comes to emotional expression: internalizers, externalizers, and those who are a "mixed bag." Those who are a mixed bag tend to lean towards either internalizing or externalizing. Even internalizers will have external behaviors associated with their emotions, they are just much more subtle than those of the externalizer.

A person's micro-culture (family) and macro-culture (culture at large) shape how a person behaves when experiencing emotions. These boundaries and limits bring a culture effectively to the "lowest common denominator" of what is tolerated. Children who are victims of interpersonal trauma usually come to the attention of others because they do not fit into the norms for age appropriate emotional expression and associated behaviors.

There are countless examples of adult women who endure years of various kinds of domestic abuse and are able to keep up a cheerful front to friends and family. Unless the woman suffers a physical injury that is visible to others, her interpersonal trauma experiences and resultant emotions may remain hidden for a long time. Experience tells me that there are many children who are likewise abused that have learned the cultural norms well enough to be able to hide their trauma experiences through emotional control in very effective ways. Some of these children may be hidden from view for years, or even decades. But some of them can only fake it for so long before the emotions come pouring out in a flood of difficult behaviors.

Thus, "emotional regulation" becomes a two edged sword: on the one hand keeping in the negative emotions under a tight rein keeps the child *looking normal* (but feeling estranged), and on the other letting loose the negative emotions as stress release that will likely result in social rejection. Clearly, the goal is to help the child to process the trauma emotions in productive ways, and to give them skills to understand and effectively address cues and triggers when they arise.

Children who have experienced abuse that has resulted in post traumatic stress behaviors have a right to be angry. How arrogant and foolhardy to aggressively work at extinguishing that rage! Any approach that targets emotional regulation as a primary or singular objective to control resultant PTSD behaviors and uses purely behavioral techniques to do this is doomed to failure.

The Gentling Approach addresses emotional regulation through what is essentially a cognitive-behavioral approach, with the "cognition" part being an educational process of didactics concerning the child learning how to adjust reactivity to response, making adjustments to erroneous attributions, and *repeated positive experience*. The "behavior" part includes not only the child's behaviors attended to by a healthy structure and boundary, but also by *how the clinician behaves with the child*.

7 Gentling and Treatment Objectives

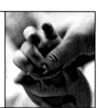

This chapter will revisit the treatment objectives, with more specific cues on what vocal characteristics and countenance approaches to use for particular objectives and situations. The reader should be apprised that while these specific approaches have been identified by in the field use with stress-disordered children, each child, situation, and clinician are unique, so your results or particular efforts may look slightly different. The following are *suggestions*. The individual clinician will need to "learn" each child and gently experiment with the suggestions in different situations to see what works best with a particular child. The major prescription is to be gentle in everything you do with the stressed child!

Lowering Physical and Psychological Agitation and Reactivity

An important first step in lowering a child's allostatic processes is to identify the often subtle behavioral "tells" that the child has. These subtle, early behaviors are keys to preventing unnecessary full-blown stress reactions. One fine strategy upon first receiving a case is to be able to visit the classroom before the child knows who you are. Even when this is not an option, classroom visits are an ideal place to begin to observe the early behavioral signs of stress.

These signs can indeed be subtle. I have observed children who bite their lower lip, or begin to bite their fingernails, or begin to touch their face, nearly every time before they begin to enter a full-blown stress episode. Fortunately, there are usually more that one of these subtle behaviors that will telegraph that the child's stress is rising. A teacher or even an aide assigned to work with the child could quite easily overlook the behaviors.

A criterion then needs to be set as to how many, how often, and what intensity will the behaviors be presented by the child before an intervention is made. There are no magic criteria for this, only good old close behavior counts and experiment-ation will indicate when it is best to intervene in order to avoid a stress episode. The idea is, of course, to make an intervention at a point when it will be most effective: before the child escalates into a stress episode. Interventions at this point are by their timing much more gentle than interventions that may need to be used at a later point.

All such interventions should make use the voice tones and countenance approaches mentioned earlier. The adult making the intervention might specifically use a neutral tone of voice, with a simple directive to the child. Remember to approach the child within their sight line; do not come up behind the child unawares, as this could trigger a strong startle reflex that is very undesirable. Also, do not stand *over* the child, but squat or kneel down beside them to talk (don't "get in their face").

The second stage of the intervention is then to give a specific directive. Here the adult making the intervention has several choices, but the main idea is to distract the child from their stress and help them to lower it to a significant degree. Again, different children may have different things or behaviors that do this for them. One seven-year-old girl brought into school a particular doll that she used to "go talk with" when the stress behaviors were noted. This seemed to calm her enough to avoid a full-blown episode.

Other ideas can be to take walk, or to take a note to the school secretary from the teacher, or to go to the library to read a book. The same principles apply in the home or community. The reader should be aware that some children will not cooperate with this "stress break" if there is not a specific task (such as taking the note to the secretary). It will also be noted that if the child resists this kind of intervention, it is likely that it was not initiated soon enough in the stress reaction cycle.

A third stage of this intervention could be gently and directly speaking with the child about the observed stress. It is not advisable to initially tell the child about those subtle behavioral signs, because this may alter the useful presentation, but simply noting that you thought the child might be a bit stressed. "It looked like you had something on your mind", or "You seemed to be getting worried, anxious, stressed, mad," etc. This helps the child to bring their stress reactivity into their consciousness, which is a fine first step in helping them to gain self-control over it.

When possible, there should be an arranged location that can be used in the school to invite the child to go to when they appear to be headed for a larger stress episode. This not only lessens disturbances in the class, but provides appropriate privacy for the child. Once again, the key is to get this invitation made and start moving out of the classroom area before the child has started to escalate. In most cases, if this is not done early enough, the child will simply refuse to leave the classroom. School staff often needs extra explanations about why the child needs to leave the class earlier than seems necessary to them.

Remember that it is human nature and nearly impossible not to become stressed yourself when someone else is highly stressed. This emotional contagion probability needs to be foremost in your mind in order to attend to yourself and gain a firm hold on your own emotional response and accompanying behaviors. There are people who just should not work in emergency situations because they cannot control their own emotional and behavioral reactivity. This makes any selection of a Therapeutic Staff Support person or school staff aide that will work daily with the child very important.

Most children respond favorably at some point in the stress episode to physical approach intended to comfort. Of course, knowing the child's abuse history is critical in this effort, because having the child interpret your physical approach as a threat would be counterproductive. With children who have been sexually abused by coercive adults, it takes more time for the child to gain trust that when you speak gently and come close, you are not trying to have sex with them.

Timing is essential in asking the child if you can come closer. You certainly do not want to do this when the stress episode is on the rise, or at the peak. In most children, there is a clear drop of physical and emotional agitation that marks the "drop" from the peak of the agitation. Some children may just sit and stare or pout. Some may begin to self-harm, while others may begin to cry or get sleepy.

When the time is right, simply *ask permission* with a kind, firm voice to step nearer or sit nearer to the child. If the child says: 'No', don't get closer! If the child does not say anything, I take the silence as a 'Maybe', and move closer. The key is not to press the physical space too quickly.

For example, if you are ten feet away from the child, don't rush forward and embrace the child when the child agrees to let you come closer. This is likely to re-trigger the stress reaction. Instead, just get closer by *half* the space. Since each child is unique, don't be surprised if even this causes the child to trigger again.

If this happens, you now have an important piece of information for the next attempt. The idea is to keep dividing the distance by half, until the child allows you to sit next to them, within actual physical contact range. Over repeated experiences of this approach should allow the child to be comfortable in allowing you get close with just one request (at the correct time, that is!)

Do not mistake that the child is "out of" their agitated state fully or completely, even if they are allowing you to sit next to them. They are simply at a different stage of the agitation than when they were aggressive or self-harming. The child may still be quite "out of it", and even in a dissociative state. Since the goal at this point is to help the child through this painful event, any admonitions or conversations are not appropriate (or productive), so resist the urge to "process" the event. Rather, in your kindest, gentlest voice and countenance, vocalize what *you see* is going on with the child. I find that using the child's name, and speaking in the third person, for some unknown reason, is quite effective.

Case Study: Laura

Laura is a seven year old girl in foster care. She has a long history in her short life of being sexually and physically abused by multiple adults. She is assigned to a part time special education classroom. Upon arrival at the school to do behavioral observations on Laura in her classroom, the clinician finds Laura and her TSS in the special education classroom in a situation of escalation.

Laura is clearly upset. Her face is flushed, her pupils are dilated, and she is cursing like a sailor. The TSS and teacher are attempting to give her firm directives to sit down, but Laura refuses. She does, though, clearly note the arrival of the male clinician in the room. This is likely due to her heightened vigilance to possible danger.

The clinician signals to the other adults to cease their efforts. The clinician then finds a chair to sit in, some distance from Laura, who is standing in the back of the classroom. Laura has a chance to catch her breath as the other adults back away from her. In a gentle, quiet, but firm voice, the clinician asks Laura if she would like to take a walk outside of the classroom. Laura shakes her head "no".

The clinician waits a moment, and then, with the same tone of voice, states (to Laura, not the other adults): "Laura seems very upset right now. She looks like she might be angry. Or frightened? I wonder which one it is." Laura shouts: "Angry!"

The clinician again waits a few moments in silence, and asks Laura once again if she would like to leave the classroom together for a walk to the designated location for Laura's privacy. This time, Laura heads for the door. Keeping reasonable distance from Laura, the clinician follows, as does the TSS.

Upon arrival at the school counselor's office, just a short distance down the hall, Laura immediately gets on the floor and crawls behind a couch in the counselor's office. The TSS begins to give Laura a directive to get out from behind the couch and sit on the couch, but the clinician blocks this, allowing Laura to hide behind the couch. In fact, the clinician asks Laura if he can sit on the floor next to the couch. Laura agrees. Again, the clinician stays silent for a few moments. Laura begins to take her shoes off (a noted sign of her stress episodes). The clinician ignores this. After a full two to three minutes, the clinician states: "That is a good hidey-place. I'll bet it feels safe in there." Laura nods: 'yes'. The clinician then asks: "I wonder if there is enough room for me back there. I like good hidey-places too." Laura pushes the couch out a bit for the clinician to be able to get behind it.

The clinician notes that Laura's face and chest flush are gone, and her face has regained some animation. He then begins to talk to Laura about how it must be very frightening and painful when Laura has these episodes. He notes that when he says this, Laura's head snaps up, and she gives him intense eye contact.

The clinician at first is concerned that this reaction may be due to his gentle voice; that Laura has misinterpreted his advance as a possible sexual threat. But he then notices that her face is animate, and she states in a very low voice, almost a whisper: "Yes, it is. How did you know?" The clinician instantly knows that he is on the right track, and the stress episode is decreasing.

The preceding example may seem quite indulgent and counter-intuitive to clinicians who have used only behavior modification techniques in the past. Many adults, even clinicians, cannot overcome the emotion and thoughts of this approach as being overindulgent or that the child is simply manipulating. But once again, the crux of the matter is the *source* of the child's upset.

This child was not being oppositional in the classic sense. She was in a defensive mode due to her trauma history. The contrast between straight behavior modification approaches and the Gentling approach is stark: in the past, with behavior modification, Laura would spend a whole day in a stressed state, getting little or no school work in. This episode using the Gentling Approach took about forty minutes from initiation to return to the classroom and ready to work.

There is no appreciable difference in the approach to stress episodes if it is used in the home or community, but the effectiveness and progress will be impaired if the child is continuing to reside in the location that their abuse occurred in, and have contact with their perpetrator. The method can be taught quite easily by modeling and direct teaching to any adult, with the exception of those adults who cannot overcome their thoughts and emotions that such a method is overindulgent, or that the child's stress reaction behaviors are disrespectful and directed at the adult.

Helping the child to feel safe again

This is a treatment objective that is usually slow to attain. The hope is to help the child to feel safe in *all environments*. It is, of course, complicated by the fact that some children may still be living or visiting in environments where their trauma took place. Hopefully, at least the perpetrator has been removed from the child's environment, and the child is not forced to have contact with their perpetrator. This complication is discussed in a later chapter dedicated to educating other serving helpers.

A second complication is that young victims have multiple and undefined cues and triggers in the forms of situations and locations. While a child may not have any reactivity in the school gym or cafeteria, they may be triggered by enclosed places such as the "reading tent" or the toilet stall. Once again, this is where concerted efforts at close behavioral observation will begin to pay off in determining likely triggers for stress episodes.

Helping a child (or anyone) to feel safe is a rather difficult task because "feeling safe" includes so many components. In addition, each person has a unique idea of what feeling safe entails. If you had to give a list of what makes you feel safe, what would your list include? A traumatized child's list will be as different as each child is from another, but some useful things can be generalized:

Components of Safety

- Firm, stable, trustworthy and caring attachments to others.
- Clear, available, healthy, and simple means for escape, if needed.
- A firmly differentiated self.
- Repeated experience of safety in different environments.
- Abandoning generalization of trauma experiences.

Interpersonal trauma really messes up a person's sense of stability and trust in other people. If this one person can so severely impact my life, what about other people? After all, the world is full of people! Re-establishing stable, trustworthy and caring attachments to adults argues for methods that encourage such progress. It is just common sense that when a child has been traumatized by abuse, a gentle approach is indicated.

Unfortunately, simply *telling* someone that you are trustworthy doesn't work; they of course have to experience you over a period of time. The same holds true of environments. If a child was locked in a closet by perpetrator, simply telling them that the toilet stall is safe will not make the toilet suddenly non-triggering.

The triggering of stress memories and subsequent reactions in situations or locations similar to the original critical incident may be able to generalize; that is, the situation or location is no longer simply a trigger for a memory, but becomes incorporated into the fabric of reactivity in its own right. Such an effect also can develop with *people*. For example, the teacher who's loud and demanding voice reminds the child of their perpetrator's countenance may become not just a cue to a memory of the abuse, but be generalized into a perceived perpetrator by the child. The effect of a child so easily generalizing situations, locations, and people as possible threats likely has its roots in the fact that children are in a stage of development that is strongly mythical and magical.

It is only through repeated, successful experiences of interpersonal trust and exposure to environments that the child will begin to feel safe with others and in diverse locations. The key to attaining the objective is to *pair* a trusted adult with environments that the child needs to function in. In order to help the child feel safe in all environments, supported experiences in different locations will include repeated reassurances by the trusted adult while in the selected environments. Rather than *stating* to the child that they are safe in a particular place, the trusted adult helper would state that they will *be with* the child in the environment, and *are ready to help* the child if needed.

Case Study: Rodney

Rodney is an eight-year-old boy who had been beaten severely by his father about a year before. His mother had left Rodney's father soon afterwards. Rodney has had problems in his classroom; he has a male teacher who tends to speak loud and forcefully. Rodney has recently been wandering out of line when he is with his class in the hallway, and when he is directed by the teacher to get back in line, he literally runs away, and out of the school building to his home, a few blocks away.

Rodney has been assigned a female aide to help keep him safe, and to help end the runaway behavior. Within the first few days of working with Rodney, the aide found a quiet moment with him and stated to him: "I know someone has hurt you very badly in the past. It is probably hard to trust other people. I will not hurt you. But you will have to watch me very closely so that you can begin to believe that." She repeated this several times over the next few days. She then had a talk with Rodney about his feelings of needing to run away when in the hallways. She theorized that Rodney might be able to control his urge to run if he was at the end of the line, and she could walk beside him. She passed the idea by Rodney, who agreed to try the suggestion. The method worked, and the aide noted after about a week that Rodney reached out and took her hand whenever the teacher raised his voice in the hallway. At that point, whenever Rodney reached out for her hand, the aide whispered to Rodney: "There goes Mr. Krill again, doesn't his voice sound loud in the hallway when he gives direction to the class?"

The reader will note that the aide used her increasingly trusted relationship with Rodney to *suggest* and *plan with* Rodney on how to address his behavior following an implicit acknowledgement of the likely source of his reactivity. Such inclusion in the treatment plan is a trust-developing tool. Rodney then spontaneously takes the aide's hand as a sign of trust and request for needed support when the teacher speaks in the hallway. Each time Rodney is able to tolerate the loud voice of the teacher, he takes one-step closer to feeling safe with the teacher in the hallways. Rodney eventually abandoned not only his generalization of reactivity to the hallways, but also to the teacher. Now, imagine if the aide was instructed to use a more classic behavior modification approach with Rodney, say, taking a "point" away each time he started to move out of line?

Affording clear, available, healthy, and simple means of escape does not necessarily refer to literal escape, though it can mean that. When the child begins to feel intolerable stress in a situation or location, they need to be able to have an acceptable way to 'escape'. In Rodney's case, he was able to hold hands with his aide. If this had not been adequate, the aide could have arranged for Rodney to squeeze her hand as a signal that Rodney needed to leave the situation in order not to enter into a full blown run away stress reaction. The use of "stress breaks" is a means to allow the child to escape situations that are strongly cueing and triggering. Eventually, the objective is to help the child tolerate such cues and triggers, thus depriving them of their power over the child's behaviors. But in the beginning for treatment, the child should be allowed this important tool to help them cope positively with their stress load.

Helping the child differentiate

The effects of interpersonal trauma are devastating to a child's sense of self identity and ego integrity. The trauma can severely damage the healthy process of differentiation that goes along with normal development. The definition of differentiation here is borrowed from Dr. David Schnarch: the ability to hold on to yourself in close intimate contact with another person. Though Schnarch's work focuses on committed adult relationships, his expanded (from Bowen) ideas about differentiation and intimacy fit very well with the needs of traumatized children.

When abuse occurs, the victim is then bound to the perpetrator in a powerfully intimate fashion. This intimacy is, of course, very sick, but intimacy does not have to be pleasant (hand to hand combat is witness to that truth). Such sick intimacy serves to fuse the victim and perpetrator in a life-long memory, if not a lifelong stunting of the victim's ability to continue to grow emotionally and psychologically.

Each time that the victim is exposed to the perpetrator, or a cue and trigger of their trauma, they are not able to 'hold on to themselves'; they are overwhelmed with the reality of their critical event and the violation of their ego integrity by their perpetrator. When the cycle of stress reactivity and stress episodes repeats and repeats, the victim is less and less able to resist being overwhelmed by the intrusive memories of the trauma. This in turn may serve to position them to become repeated victims of either the original perpetrator, or a lifelong string of perpetrators.

Successful perpetrators are successful because they have a developed skill to recognize weak and damaged will in others. They press the victim emotionally, overwhelming first their ability to hold on to their own emotions and ego structure. Then they move in for the physical or sexual abuse. A well differentiated individual is much harder for a perpetrator to engage, and thus much harder to position for abuse.

Many stress-disordered children feel this ego integrity breech keenly, and develop a strategy to guard against interpersonal trauma from reoccurring. They become "control obsessed". This control obsession can demonstrate in a variety of unhealthy ways: the child may become very internally focused, hypervigilant, or scrupulous in their manner. Or, the child becomes externally focused, gaining control of their surroundings, situations, and other people with highly agitated, aggressive, and self destructive behaviors. Stress disordered children have, by necessity, become experts at control; it's just that their control skills are designed to keep perpetrators at bay, and this skill set is not functional elsewhere.

Healthy differentiation shapes healthy control skill sets, helping children to reclaim themselves. This in turn serves to ease feelings of vulnerability, and increases a genuine sense of safety. Clinicians and caregivers need to provide strong and *repeated* messages about the child's rights to choose or refuse who and how to touch, that their private belongings (including their body) are *theirs* to choose whom to share with. (And then tolerating and supporting the child when they choose not to share.) Giving the child age appropriate opportunities to form some of their own boundaries and limits strengthens differentiation.

The right of a person to disagree or to say "no" is essential in developing healthy differentiation. Caregivers should make a habit of creating opportunities daily for a child to exercise age appropriate freedom of choice. This can be done in very simple ways: a clinician can ask the child if they would like to go to the school library or the counseling office for a talk-time, or the home caregiver might ask the child if they want their bath before or after dinner.

Because children in general feel compelled to answer an adult in a pleasing manner, they may be cooperative even when they would choose otherwise if they were free to. This effect is especially true for abused children. In my kindest voice, I often use clear *requests* instead of *directives,* and tell a child that they are free to refuse the request *with no repercussions.* There are, of course, times when directives need to be given, but use of choice should always be considered as an appropriate possible first choice.

The right of a person to openly ask for a need to be met is also essential in developing differentiation. It is not uncommon for children who have been in abusive and neglected situations to continue a habit of "stealing" food or other items to hide and eat or use in secret. These children also often do not ask for adult help when they need it, even with simple things like tying a shoe. For many, it has been much safer *not* to ask the adults in their lives for help with something, because it draws attention to the child.

Stealing and hiding behaviors in stress disordered children should not be confused with the moral issues of stealing, because their behaviors are not genuine theft, but expressions of a continued sense of not being safe and appropriately cared for. Clinicians may need to make this truth very explicit and repeat the message several times for foster parents and biological parents.

Addressing the stealing and hiding behaviors rests in being straightforward and non-punitive with the child when the items are discovered, along with *repeated demonstrations of availability of needed food and other items*. How this is done has some fine points: it is probably best if the caregiver does not call the child to the area where the food or items were found, and they should not simply remove the food or items from the hiding place and say nothing. In both of these approaches, there is a risk of triggering the child into a stress episode, because they may think that they are going to be punished.

A better way is to go to where the child is, and gently *observe:*

"I noticed that there was a peanut butter sandwich under your bed pillow. I was wondering why it was there, then I decided that maybe it is because you want to be sure to save some food in case we run out. But you don't have to worry about running out of food here, we always have enough to eat. Now, could you go get the sandwich and either eat it, or put it in a bag in the refrigerator, or throw it out if it is too old and stale?"

While there will need to be some control over a child's possible overindulgence by the caregivers, they can make healthy foods freely available at any time. One therapeutic foster parent I am fond of tells me she spends a good deal of money each month on fresh fruit that always sits in a large bowl on her kitchen counter...and I've seen the brood of children there eagerly munch on it when they come in the door after school!

This *process* of an adult caregiver offering choice and reassurances of adequate supplies of food to the child *repeatedly* provides opportunity for the adult to demonstrate deep respect for the child's ego integrity. This is a person-building interaction that the child may have either limited or no experience with. With choice comes control. With control and plenty comes safety.

Self-Initiation of Learned Stress Reduction Techniques

Since stress reactivity is a learned behavior, it makes sense that a child can un-learn it. Ideally, the child will learn how to both block and manage stress; blocking automatic reactions to triggers, and managing stress so that it does not interrupt their life quite as much. The steps in this process are to give the child the skills they need to pay attention to their own body, then process, and then self initiate stress reduction.

The first step, helping the child to become sensitive to their own physical reactivity when cued, is one that takes time and patience, because not only is every child unique in their potential for insight, but the child's age also impacts the work. With children about the age of five and older, the clinician can make much more use of cognitive restructuring type efforts that use at least a bit of logic and verbal interchange. If the child is under the age of five, the clinician then will work more heavily with the adult caregiver of the child to affect self awareness of the stress.

With all children, regardless of age, once again the meta-messages that adults give to the child are the vehicle to help the child to become self aware of their stress reactivity. By use of a gentle countenance and gentle but direct and firm language and voice tones, the child is brought to notice their stress reaction pattern and stress symptoms in a manner that is not threatening. The large message is that the child's stress reactivity is not something that is to be punished, but rather, healed.

The child is told with the adult's behavior as well as explicitly: "there is a better way to deal with your stress and interact with the world." While their resultant behaviors towards themselves, others, or belongings may be unacceptable, their illness is acceptable. Resulting difficult behaviors are *responded to* rather than *reacted to*. The child is essentially being re-educated or re-patterned, if you will, regarding how they interact with the world.

A clinician can train a caregiver to begin to notice the child's more subtle stress signs that lead up to a full-blown stress episode. Careful and close observation of the child by the clinician in multiple settings will reveal the list of small "tells" in the child's behavior that are precursors to the advance of a stress episode. If the caregiver can learn to recognize these, they can also learn how to respond to them when they see them.

The response to these early warning sign behaviors is threefold: gently observing to the child that you believe that they are becoming stressed, attempting to redirect the child to another, possibly self soothing activity, and providing the child with a firm and nurturing "ego wrapping" assist. This step may look like this:

With a gentle, calm, and moderate voice tone: "Hi there, Ralph, I see your knee bouncing. I wonder if that means we should take a break from this and take a walk?" Ralph shakes his head 'yes' and stands up to go for a walk. On the walk: "Walking feels good, even when I don't have a place that I am going to. Walking helps me to calm down. I like walking with you. You are a nice walking partner, Ralph!"

While continuing to provide the child with firm nurturing through your presence and loaned ego strength, the effort moves into speaking with the child about the details of what it is that they are feeling inside their body. This then is attached to speaking about what it is that they were thinking about when the feelings began. This processing might look like this:

With the same countenance as above: "When my knee bounces, that usually means I have big feelings inside. I wonder what big feelings you have inside you right now?" Ralph just shrugs his shoulders. "Sometimes my big feelings start when I am thinking about something that has happened to me or when I think of someone." Pause. "I wonder what you are thinking about?" Ralph begins to talk about the fact that he is worried about his little sister, who still lives in the biological home.

The next step is to help the child process the intrusive thoughts and the effect that they had on the child's body and resultant behaviors. This effort might look like the following:

"That does sound like a big worry. I'll bet it is hard to do the things you are supposed to do when you are worried like that." Ralph nods 'yes'. "That would make my knee bounce, too." Ralph nods 'yes' again. "Let's see if we can make a phone call so you can talk to your sister when we are finished with our walk. Do you think that would help?" Ralph nods 'yes'.

In separate sessions from the direct interventions on the stress signs, the next step is to teach the child methods of self-soothing that allow the child to remain in the context of where they are at. Those sessions might look like this:

"Ralph, do you remember those big feelings of worry that happen to you?" Ralph whispers "yes". "I would like to teach you how to help them like the walks help them. But I am going to teach you how to 'take a walk' without even moving away from your desk." Ralph's eyes widen in surprise. "Yes, you can make the big worry into a smaller worry, so that you can finish your math and get good grades."

At this point, any chosen method for teaching a fairly rapid physical relaxation or cognitive restructuring could be used, as long as it is age-appropriate. The reader will undoubtedly have knowledge, if not experience in teaching these to children. Since Ralph is aged seven, I might make use of my small, portable galvanic skin resistance toy to help Ralph learn to relax his body and mind through biofeedback.

I may also help Ralph to set up a process of self-talk that is positive about his sister's safety. Lastly, I would be sure to make other adults in Ralph's life that he may make use of this self calming method while he is with them, and they should be able to recognize when he is self initiating, and give him explicit permission to use the technique.

The last step is to help the child chain the entire process and to self-initiate the process on their own. At first, of course, this is with the firm and gentle coaching of the adult helper or caregiver. The 'coaching' then fades to simple presence. Encouragement and confidence in the child presented by the adults who are helping the child will eventually bring the child to a point where they can self-initiate the process and independently see it through to a self -calmed state.

While treatment is trying to "gentle" the child's here and now life experience, it should not be at the exclusion of all stress or all caution. The child still needs to have a level of normal stress that is functional in responding to directives and in keeping the child safe from further abusive situations. In most cases, this it is not an issue to mistakenly "over relax" a child's stress level or appropriate caution around strangers. But with some children who are victims of abuse, especially those who have been neglected or have been sexually abused multiple times, the child may actually *need* to be taught (if not to have a bit of healthy anxiety) to self initiate stranger caution behaviors.

Resumption of Here and Now Development

Interpersonal trauma puts a person's life on 'hold'. Everyday tasks, let alone developmental tasks become heavy burdens. Personal development slows to a crawl, because the specter of the trauma haunts every waking (and sleeping) moment.

If the clinician follows enough cases of children with PTSD, they will begin to notice how "regressed" the child seems to be, even when they are not in an active stress episode. This is most apparent when the child is observed in a larger group of peers: the child will be clearly quite socially awkward: there may be a lack of social initiation skills, or 'getting along with' skills. Other children, while perhaps not teasing or mean, seem to avoid the child. In the classroom, the child may impulsively shout out at inappropriate times, suck their thumb, or crawl under their desk. They may even begin to act like a dog or a cat. (This last behavior is consistent enough in my experience with abused PTSD children as to qualify as a marker for the disorder for me.)

Clearly, these regressed behaviors are not only making the child stand out as odd to others, but represent a stalled developmental progress. When an accurate history can be gained, this is quite valuable in then helping to direct treatment. If the child's trauma largely took place during say, their second and third year of life, and the child is now age eight, the clinician can begin to theorize that the child has missed (or at least has impairment of) about five years of some very important developmental material.

A naive clinician may simply view the regressed behaviors and begin treating them with standard behavior modification techniques with very limited success. The informed clinician will immediately understand that what is needed is to *feed the need* that the behaviors are representing. When this is done, the child becomes "full" and begins to re-take hold of his or her own growth. It's hard to complete math problems or focus on making your bed when you are starving for nurturance.

So, the first task becomes getting the adult caregivers of the child on board in understanding the reason for the regression and then the process of feeding the need.

Feeding the needs means increasing nurturing, as mentioned in the section on creating an environment of high nurturance. Another strategy in this area of treatment is to engaging the child in kinds of play that they may have not gotten enough of or have outright missed. This may be such things as playing peek-a-boo, gentle wrestling on the floor, building blanket "forts" in the living room, or playing dress-up. By "engagement", I mean literally *participating* through demonstration and shared play with the child. This might look like this:

Playfully to Samantha, age eight: "Hey Samantha, I have an idea, let's take this blanket and make a hidey-place!"

Samantha responds: "No, that's for little kids."

Bill counters: "Well, I'm going to make a hidey-place, and I'm not a little kid." Bill proceeds to start work with the blanket, with a bit of awkward acting as if he cannot get the blanket to stay put.

Samantha speaks up: "That won't work, here, let me show you!" Samantha begins to help with the hidey-place.

When it is finished, Bill crawls inside, and states: "Now, no one can see me. I'm invisible." Samantha crawls in, and states that maybe it would be nice to have some cookies in the hidey-place. Bill agrees, and both get permission from Samantha's foster mother to get some cookies.

Other demonstrations of nurturing related to the age the child was when they were traumatized could be extra cuddling, chicken-soup-type care when they are sick, and extra attention and Band-Aids® when they get scrapes and bruises. Don't forget the pouring on of daily hugs and pats on the back. It is important to note that the level of this kind of feeding may genuinely feel excessive (if not outright tiring) to the daily caregiver. While it is tiring (and the caregiver needs support), it is not excessive. Filling up the child's hunger for nurturing is not indulgent; it's feeding a starving child. Here is how it might look:

Joie, age six, falls and skins her knee at the play park while the clinician and the TSS are with her working on peer social interaction. The clinician sees the fall, and knows that one characteristic of Joie is that she has developed both emotional and physical numbing to cope with her abuse history. The clinician immediately rushes to Joie, despite the fact that she is not crying at all.

With clear concern and with a moderately loud voice: "Oh my, oh my, you are bleeding! Let me help you to the bench." To the other adult caregiver, the clinician shouts to get the first aid kit from the clinician's car. "That must hurt!" says the clinician. Joie nods "no". "Oh my, I have had a skinned knee and it stings!" the clinician counters. The first aid kit arrives, and the clinician dons gloves and proceeds to clean the wound and bandage it. Joie visibly flinches when the antiseptic wash is applied, and she says, "Yes, that does sting." The clinician looks at her and states, "Yes, it does." Joie scampers off to play again with her friends.

Robert, age ten, has had a very bad time on his visit to his biological home. There was no heat in the house, and the only toilet was not working properly. He looks sad and stressed. The foster mother invites him to sit next to her on the couch after dinner. Robert sits close, and tips his head to the foster mother's shoulder. She takes this opportunity to gently run her fingers through his hair. Robert settles in closer, enjoying the comforting feeling of being mothered.

The second task is to insist on positive movement and demonstration of age normative expected development. Again, the daily caregiver of the child may need to be educated about what is age normal for the child. It is most helpful if this adult can be given a specific and detailed list of age normal behaviors to expect of the child.

Caregivers also will likely need to be taught methods of approaching and teaching the child in the press to get the child to live up to the expectations. Caution must be exercised so as not to press so hard that the child experiences excessive stress that would spark a stress episode. The coaching process to move the child to engage in the desired age appropriate behaviors should be based both in positive approach and on expanding the child's strengths. It might look like this:

To Roger, age eight: "I see that you are a pretty strong boy when you carry your laundry basket to your room for Mom." Roger stops and flexes his bicep proudly. "I wonder if you are a big enough boy to learn how to fold and hang the clothes up. Here, let me show you how I fold a T-shirt." Roger imitates the clinician in folding. "Wow, you *can* do it! You did it a little different than I do, can you show me how you made your folds?"

The balance of feeding the needs that the regressed behaviors represent and the press for the child to behave in ways that demonstrate age normal development needs close attention, lest the balance be lost. Only feeding the nurturing needs will lead to dependence and no growth. Only work on becoming age normal will result in the child shutting down and an increase in stress episodes.

Natasha, age seven, has just calmed herself down enough by taking the foster parent's coaching to use cognitive-behavioral techniques to keep from going into a full-blown stress rage. The foster parent can now see that Natasha is simply crying in an expression of sadness, and brings Natasha her favorite doll. They hug the doll together, and the foster parent offers gentle verbalizations of empathy for Natasha's sadness. The foster parent has just paired pressure for Natasha to self-regulate her emotions in an age normal fashion *followed by* needed nurturing. There are an equal number of situations where this order might be reversed, with the nurturing coming first.

Generally, if the caregiver is attending to the details of the child's behavior, they will be able to tell if the child is at a here-and-now regressed place or an age normative place. If the child is expressing neediness for nurturing, then age normative expectations would not be pressed; the child would be attended to with nurturing instead. Once again, the worry for adults may be that the child will use a "neediness act" to avoid the age normative exercises.

But once again as well, I have faith that *a child's natural impulse is to learn, and grow towards age normal development.* If the child suddenly presents as helpless and needy, I will feed that need as a possible sign that the expectation for age appropriate behavior may have cued and triggered the child towards a stress episode, and then return to the press for age normative demonstration with support and encouragement. **Here is how that might go:**

> Shayla, age four, has been directed to pick up her toys before dinner. She has ignored the directive twice already. The caregiver approaches Shayla and asks for eye contact, which Shayla gives. She is directed again to pick up the toys, or there will be no dessert. Shayla begins to cry. Since the caregiver knows that food issues have been a trigger in the past for Shayla, she kneels in front of Shayla and states: It looks like you need a hug." Shayla accepts the hug, and begins to calm. The caregiver pulls back a bit and states: "I know that you are a big girl, and can pick up the toys. I have seen you do it before. I will sit right here and watch you pick them up. Then we can have supper *and* dessert!" Still whimpering a bit, Shayla begins to pick up the toys.

The wise caregiver attended to both the need for support and nurturing, and held the age normal expectation. The caregiver does not jump to the conclusion that needy and regressed behaviors *always* represent avoidance of an undesired task or manipulation. Careful discernment is the key.

Experiencing of Positive Re-engagement

Certainly all of the aforementioned specific examples of carrying out Gentling demonstrate positive re-engagement of a child who has been abused and has PTSD as a result. However, I would like to offer a few comments about the *quality* of engagement that I feel is a fundamental aspect to the Gentling process.

Victims of interpersonal trauma have experienced a horrendous kind of engagement with their perpetrator. There may be multiple perpetrators, helping to force a quicker generalization of mistrust and dysfunctional, reactive style of engagement with others. For many children who are victims of repeated neglect, physical and sexual abuse, there is also a long history of intergenerational family chaos. Their primary relationship engagements are mostly all negative in *quality* as well as volume. Any clinician who has had the chance to work inside the homes of such families will immediately understand the overwhelming sensation of sitting in the midst of such illness. These homes often have continual and unrelenting hostility, resentment, unfulfilled needs, aggression, frustration, drama, and fusion. In short, they are extremely undifferentiated. These children are in sore need of positive engagement, which, of course, is not easy: the child may be so used to negative engagement, that they genuinely do not know how to engage positively.

If Gentling is used only as a *technique,* I do not feel that it is as effective as if the helper has genuinely bought into the approach. If Gentling is only a technique, the helper may not be able to "hold on to themselves" when the child stubbornly continues to engage negatively, despite the helper's use of the "technique". I have to believe that there is a salient difference between using gentleness as a technique, and consciously integrating gentleness as a *quality* of a helper's helping countenance. Gentleness accepted and used at this deeper level has a quality of intimacy that can be disquieting for the helper. Positive engagement in the Gentling approach is not for the faint of heart.

All therapeutic process is intimate for both the receiving patient and the giving therapist, even if the therapist might distance themselves from such notions. There are many therapists who are themselves quite uncomfortable with intimacy, and/or do not have a very accurate clinical view of intimacy. Certainly speaking with a child about their interpersonal abuse is a painful intimacy, one that many good clinicians would prefer to avoid. Such details are certainly intimate, not because they may have to do with sexual matters, *but because they have to do with the core of whom the victim is.*

When the child heals to a point of ego strength that allows them to differentiate enough (read: self-regulate their emotions surrounding the abuse and the processing of the details), they will be able to reveal the core of who they are, and what the trauma has done to change them. This is a very intimate act for the child: showing someone else who they really are, not just the collection of difficult behavioral stress signs. This truth implies that the processing of the trauma must *post date* the work done to build ego strength and differentiation. Without the positive engagement ability and gain of ego strength, the processing will likely have less effect, and in fact, may just re-traumatize the child. This mistake is taken up in a later chapter addressing the issue of a person being a trigger for the child

While patients revealing intimate details are certainly expected, and clinicians are certainly aware of the need for respectful and empathetic response to a patient's revelations, there usually remain varying levels of distancing that the clinician employs due to their early training as a therapeutic helper. Professional distance, as anyone who has done therapy work for while knows, is largely an intuitive process, that benefits from consistent supervision in order to remain appropriate. By its nature, the Gentling approach walks the line of emotional intimate exchange at a much closer tolerance than other forms of therapy. It needs to do this in order to ensure "breaking through" the tough shell of detachment and numbness that the child is suffering and that goes along with PTSD in children who have been victims of interpersonal trauma. Not every clinician, counselor, or foster parent is cut out for it.

As helpers, our own pain tolerance is a key in helping victims of abuse. If the helper has a low tolerance for such painful material that a child victim may present, the helper will at least unconsciously, if not consciously avoid entering into this arena with the child. Such avoidance, I believe, leads the child to an understanding that they must *protect the helper* from the gory physical and emotional details. The helper that prefers to stick with the here-and-now issues (forgetting their connection to the gory details) may offer up a positive, "feel good" engagement that will be transparently not genuine to the child. This kind of 'positive engagement' will struggle to ever be more than just a surface demonstration of a behavior set. The child is forced to hold on to the numbing and detachment, because there has not been anything viable to replace these protective tools.

Gentling seeks to "sit with" the victim in the painful, intimate, sorrowful, grieving place that lives deep inside the child. This is the start and heart of what "positive engagement" really means. The helper's job is to positively engage the pain (and details) of the trauma, not just once or twice during sessions geared towards processing the trauma history, but as a subtext to the "moving on" following the important processing and corrections of attributions.

Naive clinicians may believe that once the basic processing of the history is complete, the pain must be over. It is not, of course. Just like any grieving, it may take years for the wounds to fully heal. Even then, they will always ache intermittently. Our culture has a very low tolerance and patience for grief work. And a child victim of interpersonal abuse has much to grieve.

Though positive re-engagement is a therapeutic objective, the process of *doing* it may not appear to be all that 'therapeutic.' Casual day to day interactions that are upbeat, positive in orientation, and perhaps centered upon playfulness or actual play are all tools to meet the objective. Further, positive engagement needs to be remembered as a maintenance tool as well.

There are times when the child simply needs a break from relentless issue facing, stress behaviors, processing, and just plain bad days. My decade's long hobby of magic has served this objective very well. Having an interesting pocket trick at hand to intrigue a child's curiosity has been a fine form of positive engagement. I am sure the reader can come up with his or her own such enjoyable engagement tool.

So: positive engagement has many layers, from day to day nurturing, age normal expectations, play, fearlessly embracing the reality and details of the child's abuse history and pain, and daily support to help them live with the ache of horrible memories.

Reconnection, and Feeling Trust with Others

Beyond positive re-engagement lies the deeper layers of intimacy and trust that make life secure and worth living. People who experience trauma sometimes describe themselves as "feeling out of it", or "in a fog". Anyone who has had a sudden (or even expected) death of a loves one can readily relate to this sensation. When interpersonal trauma has occurred, connections with other people are damaged in the area of trust. Not only is the victim now suspicious of other people, they are suspicious of their own ability to assess danger and size up other people as potential threats.

The side-effect of damaged connections and ability to connect in new relationships is a profound loneliness that the victim feels. At least in war, soldiers may be able to gain the "Band of Brothers" effect, which may serve to mitigate some of the loneliness of trauma. In some cases, siblings who have experienced similar levels and types of abuse may develop (either positive or negative) intense connections between each other. But for the child who has experienced their trauma alone, they tend to live with it alone afterwards. Essentially, the child traumatized by abuse carries not only posttraumatic stress, but is taking the first steps towards human attachment problems as a reaction to the trauma.

Dysfunctional families that include neglect, sexual, and physical trauma are usually (notoriously) hostile towards helping agencies such as child protective services. By extension, they tend to be hostile as well towards other helpers like therapists. Such open hostility is quite readily transmitted to the child; the parent or caregiver may also have actually warned the child what not to say, and that the helpers are simply wolves in disguise, intent on harming the child. One of the most frequent tools used by these parents that I have encountered is that the parent tells the victimized child that if they cooperate with the helping services, the child will be separated from their siblings *forever*.

Even in treatment situations where the child is continuing to live in the care of a non-offending related adult, there may be hostility from this adult in the form of resentment towards the helpers. The adult may feel offended or insulted that they cannot manage the child alone, or are fearful that the child will be removed from them. They may have had other experiences with such helpers that ended poorly. While the adult may be judged adequate by legal standards, they may not have the motivation, insight, or even intellectual capacity to easily or adequately learn the concepts and interventions needed on a daily basis for the child to progress. On the bright side, the child victim hopefully has an established minimum of trust with this caregiver.

For some child victims, there is the problem of what I call "pseudo-trust"; some children tend to become very forward and (apparently) trusting of anyone and everyone. This is most often seen in children under the age of about seven. Most young children, as they proceed in their development have periods of "strangeness" around even extended family members. This alternates with precocious periods where the child is easily friendly with just about anyone.

Some PTSD children appear to "get stuck" in one or the other of these stages. Those stuck in the overly cautious (sometimes labeled "shy") stage are understandable; this serves as an appropriate vigilance against further abuse. Those stuck in the "pseudo-trust" stage could be mistaken by a clinician as a child fully ready to delve into their history of abuse. In most cases, they are not.

In my experience, the child who is expressing this "pseudo-trust" is simply hedging their bets, so to speak, with other people. They have likely learned at some point in their abuse that "sucking up" can be a useful technique to avoiding more abuse. Or, if they have been sexually abused, such "flirtatious" behaviors engender the interest and attention of others. All of this, of course, makes reconnection and development of trust a tall order, but not an impossible one.

It is troublesome that the emerging systems of "managed care" and foster care programs seem to bypass or even ignore the issue of trust so quickly. While people in the helping organizations readily accept that they and the foster parents are safe and can be trusted (in the sense of having training and the proper clearances), this has little meaning to a six year old child who has a history of being beaten and molested from many adults in her life. Therapists who perhaps have an inflated view of themselves to the point where they allow exactly 2.5 sessions to establish "joining" are quite similarly guilty. Trust and reconnection, worked on by creating a proper environment, given opportunity for, and shaped gently, are all guided by the pace that the *child* sets.

Consistent gentleness engenders trust. While a child's perpetrator may have demonstrated gentleness as a means to coerce or manipulate the child, perpetrators cannot maintain an honest gentleness consistently. Remember that gentleness is not a wishy-washy, Pollyanna kind of thing, but that it is firm, kind, and structured.

When consistency is added, the child is able to find the helper much more predictable in mood, affect, and behavior. This of course, is the exact opposite of what the child experienced for the perpetrator. If the perpetrator was known to the child (most are), the child likely developed a healthy mistrust and caution about the perpetrator's approach and interactions.

Many children will, in fairly quick order, begin to offer a level of trust to helpers based upon the Gentling approach. It is a wise clinician, though; who does not take this initial show of trust as one that runs very deep. If the clinician misinterprets this level of trust as something more than it is, and attempts to begin to poke into the issues of history uninvited, the child will indicate their genuine level of trust by shutting down the helper. Remember, Gentling allows the child to lead the clinician into the history, not the other way around.

It is a rare case of trauma inflicted by abuse in a child that develops the needed trust to address history under a six month time frame. Some treatments for PTSD (of course based on adult victims) claim to be able to successfully end symptoms in very short order. While this may (or may not) work for adults, applications of these methods to children do not have a proven track record, and may be more intense and damaging to tiny, fragile, or almost totally missing egos.

Furthermore, in cases where a child victim of interpersonal trauma has been placed in a foster home, they do not have just one person (like a clinician) to develop trust with, but a whole new family as well. These new relationships with foster parents, foster siblings, and all of the other helpers involved take time to sort out and develop.

And so the development of trust towards intimate reconnection is key to treating children who have been traumatized by abuse. Any good clinician has had education on how to present themselves in ways to develop trust and working relationships with patients, so I do not need to detail such steps here. In cases of childhood trauma though, the clinician needs to understand that they cannot *talk* their way into gaining trust with such children. While the clinician, of course, must speak, and may speak about trust, relying on such discussions to gain the needed trust is mistaken. Rather, trust is gained by consistent, repeated, gentle *demonstration* that the child is safe with the clinician.

There is much more to gain by repeatedly verbalizing to the child that you will "protect them, no matter what", or that they are "too precious to let get hurt", or "no one is allowed to hurt you" than, "It's OK, you can trust me, I'm a counselor."

In some more severe cases, trust development and reconnection is exceedingly slow and difficult. Not only helping systems, but also many clinicians lack the patience to work through this extended period of distrust resolution. There are several additional things that I have found to be helpful in such tough situations. First, recall what was stated earlier about 'becoming the child's age.' I have found that if I do this with the child in the context of self-revealing, even children who are very distrustful will offer me empathy. I sometimes use recollections of fearful or painful situations from my days as a child, or those that I have experienced as an adult.

To Matilda, age seven: "Sometimes I have bad dreams. I have had one bad dream that keeps on coming back, over and over. I've had it since I was about your age." Matilda asks what my dream is about. "Let me draw you a picture as I tell you about it. In my dream, I'm running really hard. I look behind me, and there is a giant, mean pickle chasing me." (This inevitably engenders a giggle from the child, as I have also just completed a cartoon of a giant, running pickle with a mean face.) I make a slight frown, and ask: "You are not making fun of my bad dream, are you?" The child always nods 'No', and usually proceeds to begin to draw a picture of his or her own bad dream. Empathy is a beautiful thing; it works both ways as a therapy tool.

Curtis, age ten, a victim of years of abuse and neglect, had found his infant sister dead in her crib. "I heard you had a sister who died. That is a hard thing. My mother died last year. Even though she was sick for a long time, when she died, I cried and cried. My Dad picked me to carry my Mom's urn from the funeral place back to his house. That was very hard for me to do." Curtis nods his understanding, the tears welling up in his eyes tell me of his empathy.

The child's gift of empathy to me builds the trust that they need to reconnect. Empathetic connection recursively strengthens trust.

Approaching and Working Through the Critical Incident

As stated earlier in this book, approach to the child's history of abuse ideally should be done very gently and at the pace that the child sets, not the clinician's, not the child protective service case worker's, and not the courts. But that, of course, is in an ideal world. There are often situations of interpersonal abuse towards a child that press for details of the abuse from the child in order to make a determination of the need for removing the child from the care of the caregiver.

These cases most often surround issues of neglect, emotional abuse, or sexual abuse. This "press" (usually by child protective services and the court) to have the child relate details of the abuse allegations has very mixed results, especially with younger children. Though I know of no reliable studies on the subject, I would state that in my experience, such "pressing" either usually ends with the child shutting down and soon being returned to the perpetrator (especially if there is inconclusive or no physical evidence), or the development of a plethora of false and confusing statements from the child (refer to the famously botched child abuse case of People vs. Buckey that took many years to come to the conclusion that no abuse took place.)

Though detailing the particulars of questioning, memory, and child protection practice concerning children as court witnesses is beyond the scope of this book, the reader will want to become familiar with these issues. In particular, a full understanding of Child Sexual Abuse Accommodation Syndrome as it applies to court proceedings would be key, as would be gaining a thorough understanding of how question-response material is accessed and potentially used in court situations. Ceci and Bruck's (1995) book on this subject, *Jeopardy in the Courtroom: A Scientific Analysis of Children's Testimony* is a classic authority on forensic concerns.

A common situation where a clinician is working with a PTSD diagnosed child victim of interpersonal abuse is when the child has been placed in foster care. In these situations, while there has been a clear determination of neglect or physical abuse, the child may begin to relate further recollections of abuse, usually to the foster patent. Especially if the child's return to the original caregiver is imminent (exposure to one or more perpetrators, but not necessarily a parent-perpetrator), getting the details of the alleged abuse from the child becomes important to the child's continued well-being and care.

The clinician once again is faced with pressures to "press" the child faster than is guided by the Gentling approach. The best the clinician may be able to do is to try and slow down those pressing for the child to reveal details, and to work hard at creating the most favorable, safe, and therapeutic relationship for the child to move into detailing their trauma. When possible, a child who has recently made revelations about abuse while in foster care should be afforded the privilege of being questioned by the child protection staff assigned to do the forensic questioning while having either the therapist or foster parent (or both) in close proximity for support. The chapter on Educating Caregivers foster, parents, teachers, child protection workers, and judges, further details guidelines and recommendations for each of these disciplines.

These typical and pervasive problems aside, the clinician will eventually be in position in treatment with a child to approach the traumatic incidents. There are several key tools to use and guide the clinician through this often difficult and painful process. If the clinician has begun to use the Gentling approach and techniques in earnest, they have already begun to *create a safe therapeutic space* between themselves and the child.

Once this space begins to produce a sense of safety and trust, the clinician needs to *be prepared for the opportunity* to more or less directly address the trauma material. In many cases, this *permission or invitation by the child* occurs through play, but it may also be more direct than that, with the child beginning to speak directly and without euphemisms about their abuse trauma.

In the case of play, the clinician does a wise thing in making *on the floor routine play* a part of their work with the child. This floor time engages the child in familiar activity, and offers plenty of opportunity to head in the direction of trauma material. Often, fantasy play with action figures or dolls becomes a euphemism for the child's trauma experience. This has seemed to me more likely so with children younger than about age seven. In many cases, the working through of the history material with young children through such allegorical, fantasy play is effective in symptom relief, and additional detail-by-detail accounting of events becomes redundant and unproductive.

Once again, the problem with such efforts is that if the child protective services and court is pressing for specific details to make a case against returning the child to the perpetrator, Kermit the Frog beating up on Batman during a therapy session is not the evidence the court needs. In such situations, I may gently ask the child if real people behave the way the action figures are behaving. If he or she says 'Yes', I would follow with "Who?" The idea is for the child to begin to have the freedom to speak about and process their wounds. While this line of questioning is not forensically focused or forensically intended, if such fact witness testimony (provided by the clinician to the court) eventually is helpful to the child in court, so much the better.

As soon as the clinician senses that trauma history material is surfacing they need to make continual *close observation of the child in the moment.* It is the child's physical response, or "body language", that will guide the clinician on whether to continue, slow down, or entirely stop pursuing trauma history material. Look for a fairly relaxed countenance to the child. Any moderate to severe agitation, either physically or emotionally is a signal to stop the process.

Likewise, if the child demonstrates a rapid dissociation effect, stop the approach. Understand that some emotional expression is acceptable and desirable, but the more esoteric signs of decompensation are to be taken seriously and avoided. Remember that there is *no gain in pushing this process beyond what the child has given permission for you to be present to. Allow the child to lead.* Putting the child into a stress episode is simply not worth it. If the child can go away from the session feeling that they are safe and comfortable despite speaking about their trauma, they will do so again at a later time. With each repeat of this safe process, they begin to heal.

It is important to note that the child may or may not show signs of physical or emotional agitation due to the material. Though many children will begin to show signs of being upset either physically or emotionally or both, a good number of children will speak about their abuse in a rather neutral, unemotional fashion indicative of detachment and numbing. Both extremes of the responses are useful as further material to work through: "It looks like talking about this gets you angry/upset/sad/feeling hurt." Or "It looks like talking about this leaves you with no feelings at all." When these behavioral signs are present (but not to the degree of decompensation), the clinician can use them to begin to sensitize the child about how the stress behavior cycle works and affects the child.

Any good clinician knows to *attend to both expressed emotion and content* at the same time. One mistake of novices is to lose balance in this effort; sometimes getting "target fascination" about the details at the expense of the child's increasing stress level in the session. Remember that the clinician's goal is healing, not gathering forensic evidence for court. It also must be kept in mind that a person's recall of trauma events is often clouded and spotty. This is especially true if the trauma took place when the person was very young. Getting accurate, detailed content is far less important (at least therapeutically) than is *giving emotional support, helping the child to feel safe,* and *correcting any mistaken attributions of responsibility* that the child has.

As mentioned in an earlier chapter, what and how *language* is used in Gentling is fundamental. The clinician's tone, volume, and content are all very important in approaching the trauma history. I have witnessed overworked, rushed and impatient child protective service caseworkers ask direct and specific questions of a young child, and watched that child "shut down" into a highly stressed and non-communicative state.

I have also been present when clinicians have done the same, and also use phrases and words far too advanced for the child's age. Children, and especially young children who have been traumatized by interpersonal abuse, often do not have the ego strength to withstand such intense cues and triggers to their trauma to be able to give the "facts" to the investigating worker, or a concise and articulated description of their symptoms to a clinician. In working with abused children with PTSD, there is not greater virtue than patience.

The more productive tactic to use once the child has given evidences of readiness to process is to use less harsh and gentler content. Using language that the child uses and understands, using some indirect content, as well as using a slow speaking pace is effective. While it is likely that the clinician already knows at least some of the details of the abuse the child has suffered from psychological and child protective reports, they should not be so brutal as to bring these up in a pointed fashion with the child. In addition, while the clinician needs to let the child know that any information about abuse must be reported, they can do this without such a blunt and cold statement.

The Gentling approach, rather, speaks of "the bad/frightening things that have happened to you" as a way of signaling to the child that the clinician knows about the trauma the child has experienced. Letting the child know that if needed, the clinician will "tell some other people who will help protect and keep you safe if someone is hurting you" is informative, fair, and gentle. Below is a vignette to illustrate these points:

Alex, age six, is playing with the clinician with action figures in a situation that Alex has set up. Currently, the Batman figure is climbing a string "rope" to get to the top of the coffee table to save Miss Piggy. Miss Piggy is being accosted by a Godzilla action figure, and Miss Piggy is screaming, "He's killing me!" Alex is playing Batman and Miss Piggy, and Alex has assigned the clinician to play "mean Godzilla."

At a pause in the play, the clinician "wonders" if real people ever do these things. The clinician notices that Alex pauses in his movements and looks down at the floor. The clinician states that is seems as if Miss Piggy was very frightened, and wonders if Alex might have had some frightening things happen in his life.

Alex nods his head, and says, almost in a whisper: "I hate it when people yell and fight." The clinician says: "Me too. It might be OK if people raise their voices when they disagree, but fighting can be frightening." Alex proceeds to relate that he had witnessed his father rape and beat up his mother. The clinician tells Alex that she will be asking for some other people to help keep Alex safe from having to go through something like that ever again. Would Alex have gotten as much therapeutic benefit if the clinician, already knowing the history, simply directly asked Alex to relate the details of the crime he witnessed?

In this clinician's experience, children generally go through a "history phase" in the treatment, meaning that they spend some time in the active processing of the critical incidents. This phase seems to last weeks or months, depending on the child, their experiences, duration, type, and frequency of abuse. The temptation for the clinician remains pressing the child beyond the time that the child wants to share history details. Some clinicians, having internalized an adult model of PTSD treatment, may believe that repetition of the sordid details is in some way helpful. While this may be true in adult cases of individuals who had a strong and mature ego structure prior to the critical incident, it is a serious question if the same holds true of abused children.

My clinical sense tells me that when the child decides to stop processing the history, it is time to stop processing the history. The theory is that the child will likely alternate their focus and energy between processing and developmental growth for some time to come; with repeated examinations (with or without a clinician) at various important times in their life.

In summary, the clinician needs to understand legal implications of trauma material that fit the description for a crime, and need to be prepared to be called to court. They need to approach their work with these things in mind, but avoid being forensically focused. The Gentling approach to a child's historical trauma material should embody a high level of respect for the child. This respect is demonstrated by allowing the child to control the pace of processing, not imposing brutal and direct questioning, never putting leading words or ideas into the child's mind, and being extraordinarily gentle with their deep and painful wounds.

8 Problems with Traditional Behavior Modification Techniques

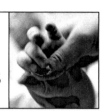

The use of traditional behavior modification techniques with stress disordered children needs to be done with caution and extra care. The issue of the *primary source* of the child's behaviors needs to take precedence over simply "pressing on" with behavior modification techniques. The key indicator to the clinical team treating the child is that they will find the child's behaviors getting *much worse*. This initially can be mistaken as an "extinction burst", and the team then may be motivated to apply more behavior modification pressure.

Of course, such efforts are doomed, because the central issue is not "non-compliance", but reactivity to stress loads. Essentially, such adherence to strict behavior modification protocols in working with PTSD children is working out of a mistaken idea of what the source of the behavior is (read: "the child is trying to manipulate, avoid work, is trying to control, or get attention.")

It is often difficult for clinicians who have a strong background (and success) with behavior modification to adapt to the Gentling Approach because it feels counter-intuitive. Not only clinicians, but teachers, Therapeutic Support Staff, parents, and foster parents also struggle with the change from a classic behavioral approach. But again, the "proof is in the pudding", so to speak: when repeated attempts to use a behavioral technique that *should* work is not working, behavior modification theory states that the plan needs to be reworked. In this case, the behavior modification techniques, though still very valuable, *must make room for the Gentling Approach to work side by side.* Indeed, there are times when the behavior modification techniques *must take a back seat* to the Gentling Approach *if progress is to be made.*

Behavior modification techniques are excellent in helping a stress disordered child to feel safer in their environment, especially if the child comes from a family of origin environment that has been chaotic and inconsistent in setting boundaries and limits. Tightening boundaries and limits adds to the security and lessens stress loads for the child. The trick is for the caregiver to know when and more importantly, *when not* to use behavior modification techniques. Essentially, classic behavior modification techniques are inherently stress-inducing. Applying them *during* a stress episode is simply counterproductive.

Secondary to this is for caregivers to be able to accurately ascertain when the child's stress levels are at the edge of the child's tolerance. Another way of expressing this is that once the child is at the "tipping point" of being near the entry into a stress episode, behavior modification techniques will only serve to push the child into the highly painful and destructive stress episode.

Overall, the application of behavior modification techniques should not be the first choice of approaches in the beginning of treatment. They grow in use, scope, and intensity as the child's stress levels decrease. Care must be taken along the way of the increase to ascertain if the selected behavioral techniques and the scope of their use is overloading the child's stress tolerance. This is not to ignore the difficult behavior issues that the child may have, and that may, in fact, be quite pressing. It's just a matter of "triage". You can't work the underlying difficult behaviors of manipulation, opposition, nastiness, and social awkwardness until the stress levels stabilize to a level that allows such work. A case example will provide the reader with clearer understanding of how traditional behavior modification methods may prove difficult with PTSD children:

Angel, Age Seven

Angel was a seven year old child who had been in her first foster home for about six weeks when I was called into the case; the foster parents were already considering passing her along to another foster family due to her intense behaviors. She had just completed a week stay in the regional children's mental health hospital because she had broken a window during a stress episode and had begun to bang her head against the wall so fiercely that it cracked the plaster. The stay in the mental health hospital did not alter any of her symptoms, just provided a respite for the beleaguered foster family. In fact, the stay ay have made things worse, since the hospital routinely physically restrained children and placed them in isolation rooms when they are upset.

Angel had experienced a wide variety of abuse when living with both of her parents, who traded she and her nine year old sister her back and forth between the divorced couple. When in their father's home, the girls were quite neglected, running the streets, often dirty, and not having enough to eat. When in their mother's home, they witnessed domestic abuse towards their mother by boyfriends, and some issues with the boyfriends making sexual advances on the girls. The mother worked as an exotic dancer, and left the girls at home at night with different unrelated males. In one of Angel's most vivid nightmares she is trapped inside a clothes dryer. This dream apparently came from the fact that Angel's older sister used to actually do this to hide Angel from the adult male sexual perpetrators in the home.

Angel and her sister were removed from the mother's care following the mother having taken both girls to Las Vegas, gotten tired of them, and then placing them on a bus to send them back to the East coast to a distant single male relative who was later identified as a known sexual perpetrator. Since the children's father was willing to take the older girl with supports offered by child protective services, but not Angel, she was placed in foster care.

The foster family, while good, salt-of-the-earth people, were having a very hard time accepting the oppositional and defiant behaviors that Angel was exhibiting. They had almost a decade of foster care experience, but had never cared for child as reactive as Angel. Most of the children they had cared for in the past were children who were able to be returned to their biological parents within a year to eighteen months. They had relied for their entire careers on the use of high standards for behavior and the use of classic behavior modification techniques that they had learned in their foster care training and from therapists in their home over the years.

Upon observing Angel and the foster parents in the home, two things became quickly clear: the foster parents were in fact using behavior modification techniques (and did this accurately and well), and Angel was entering intense, prolonged stress episodes when they used the techniques. As with most adults, the foster parents applied stronger and stronger pressure when they experienced Angel displaying opposition and defiance.

In addition to her high sensitivity to any perceived pressure coming from an adult, she also engaged in daytime wetting when in a stress episode. When the foster parents gave a directive to Angel, she would simply say 'no'. When prompted a second time, she would begin to scream and cry. When the foster parents prompted a third time, this time with a stated consequence (ten minute time out in the 'naughty chair' in the family dining room), Angel would often simply continue to cry, squat, and urinate through her clothing. The foster parents interpreted the entire sequence as direct opposition and defiance to their good efforts at care and control of the child. They related their frustration to me, stating that prior to my involvement a therapist that they highly respected and found success with in the past had advised them to increase the levels of consequence on the child, and demand that the child immediately disrobe and bathe, then clean up the urine form the floor. After hearing Angel's story, the dear, compassionate reader will understand why these measures were not only ineffective, but (unintentionally) abusive to this child.

Appealing to the foster parents in the same fashion as I have disclosed to the reader, they began to moderate their behavioral methods to only use them when Angel was clearly not in a stress episode, and to alter their basic approaches to directives to ease the level of perceived pressure by Angel. They began to identify when Angel was in a stress episode and used Gentling approaches exclusively. Following the completion of the stress episode, they returned to the behavior modification skills that they were so good at to address any misbehaviors that Angel engage in when in the stress episode.

Instead of making demands that she disrobe and clean up the floor, the foster parents began to approach the wetting incidents with gentleness and an attitude of: "oh my, sweetheart, you have had an accident, let's go upstairs with (foster parent) Mommy and have some privacy to clean up." Taken by the hand and gently led to the shower, and then afterwards, the clean up done with the foster parents' help, along with a gentle chat about Angel's emotions and how Angel might approach an adult for emotional support rather than wetting ensued. Angel did make amazing progress, and following almost two years of Gentling treatment, found a 'forever' home and family. One year following, she looked like any average, happy child.

9 Special Considerations in Sexual Trauma Cases

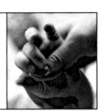

Working with a child who has been sexually abused is profoundly disturbing. While some clinicians can work with neglected or physically abused children, many just cannot find a way through their own emotions to be able to work with child sexual abuse survivors. It is important that those who find it too difficult within themselves excuse themselves from working with child sexual abuse victims. Professionals who have difficulty with the area tend to avoid any addressing of "that thing that happened to you", or they simply ignore important behavioral clues or gestures by the child, or simply treat some other diagnosis that the child doesn't even have.

For those with the courage to treat, there are some fundamental concepts that need to be understood and accepted. These truths at first seem at odds to our usual way of thinking about sexuality and children. The first truth is that children are sexual beings, even in-utero. Interestingly, adult sexual perpetrators of children appear to understand intuitively that children are sexual beings. Of course, being a 'sexual being' does not mean that their sexuality is fair game for an adult to abuse, or that their sexuality is on par with an adult's (though some adult's sexuality may be on par with a child's!)

It is fairly common knowledge that even very young children engage in sexual self stimulation at varying frequencies and intensities. Though "average" sexual behaviors in children at different ages covers a certain spectrum, most clinicians with any developmental training will understand the scope of what is expected to be seen at any particular age. As adults, even though we may know the facts of childhood sexual development and expression, we may tend to "block out" this information as being, well, uncomfortable to think about, let alone a topic to engage a child in treatment.

The point is that children are fully "wired" sexually. While their wiring lies largely dormant until developmental progress reaches a point where full sexual awakening occurs, it surely can be "powered up" when an older child or adult decides to perpetrate a sexual crime against a child. Once the psychosexual system is powered up, it is not easy to simply switch off.

This leads to a second, rather uncomfortable fact to confront: the sexual contact that the child had may have been, at least in part, or at an initial stage of the abuse, pleasant to the child. As a parent myself, and as someone who has worked with countless innocent and precious small children, this is a very difficult fact indeed to absorb. Sexual perpetrators of children will often use the existing level of intimacy in the relationship to press for sexual contact, leading the child to believe that the contact is an expression of affection and love.

The perpetrator is lying to the child. The sexual behavior has nothing to do with love or affection. The child, as a sexual being, may respond sexually to the overtures. It is only at a later time, possibly as early as during the abusive act itself, or perhaps many abuse episodes later that the child begins to experience the crushingly negative effect of the abuse.

The Touch Continuum, developed originally by Cordelia Anderson, is the program that most adults know as the "good touch-bad touch" approach to educating (and questioning) children about possible sexual abuse. What most adults do not know is that the "good touch-bad touch" is only part of what the program includes. There is a third category that Anderson uses named "confusing touch".

If educators and clinicians only teach the "good touch-bad touch" ends of the continuum, we risk communicating to children that sexual touch is "bad". While sexual touch is inappropriate and bad when an adult (or an older child) sexually touches a child sexual touch itself, of course, is not inherently "bad".

The reader will obviously see the conundrum: educating children about possible sexual abuse, or treating a child who has been sexually abused without causing (further) damage to their sexuality by labeling sexual touch "bad". It is well known that many children who have been sexually abused may engage in more frequent and intense masturbation. If I, as the clinician, speak to them about "the bad man who touched them in a bad way" without qualifying that what made the touching in the child's private areas "bad" was that the one touching was an adult, the child may receive the message that when they touch themselves sexually (or anyone does when they are an adult), they are "bad" as well.

As clinicians treating children who have been sexually abused, we must carefully weigh what and how we say things to the child. The child has been wounded not only physically, but also psycho-sexually. This complexity of sexual wounds will undoubtedly follow the child into their adolescence and adulthood. It is a grave responsibility for people treating a sexually abused child to articulate and distinguish between what the perpetrators did and what healthy sexual expression is.

The child needs to be told specifically that the perpetrator's actions were abusive, violent, tricky, and that a child cannot really consent to sex. On the other hand, the child also needs to have healthy sexuality affirmed by telling them specifically that sex between two adults who (are able, because they are adults) agree is normal, caring, loving, and not "bad".

Acknowledging that what the perpetrator did may have initially felt good and acceptable to the child, but the child was "tricked" by the perpetrator is a good place to start. By doing this, we clearly are letting the child "off the hook" so to speak regarding any pleasure that they initially felt: just because it felt good does not make it your responsibility or make you a bad child...you were tricked...it is the adult who is responsible and bad.

Sexual abuse damages a child's sense of trust and intimacy. Following the abuse, re-connection with adults in a healthy fashion may be a very confusing and difficult endeavor for them. It is not unusual for children who have been sexually abused to become "clingy" to the adults who are caring for them. This clinginess may even at times cross the line into what I call "amorous" behaviors. Alternately, the same child may have periods of time when they totally reject any kind of physical demonstration of affection or care, even flinching when an adult simply places a hand on their shoulder.

As in all cases of traumatic abuse with children, gentleness should be the guiding beacon in treatment. Being direct, using clear and specific language, and clarifying sexual abuse from healthy sexuality does not have to be harsh or pushy. On the other hand, it is perhaps in the area of sexual abuse trauma more than other kinds of trauma that the clinician must be aware that that the "gentling" approach can trigger a child who has had a perpetrator use gentle, kindly voice tones and approaches. The child may interpret our approach as seductive, like the perpetrator's. While the clinician can still remain gentle, they can raise the *volume* of their voice, and be sure to speak to the child in an open environment that the child is aware that there are other (safe) adults around.

Once the child has acknowledged to the clinician that they are a victim of sexual trauma, the clinician should make a clear and specific statement to the child that they (the clinician) will never abuse them. Note that this statement should only be made *after* the child has acknowledged abuse to the clinician. Believe it or not, I have seen other clinicians walk up "cold" to a child and begin to ask them about their sexual abuse! Since sexual abuse is such a *deeply personal violation*, such an approach is *equally deeply disrespectful to the child,* and it borders on abuse itself.

10 | An Environment of High Nurture, High Structure

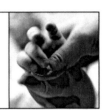

Inevitably, a number of neglected and abused children are removed from their biological family by Children and Youth Services and placed in alternate care, either waiting for legal maneuvers to end, or their parent(s) to regain enough stability and corrective parenting skills to take them back home. Children removed from traumatic, abusive situations are also inevitably being removed from a home that is either chaotic or severely dysfunctional, or both. These homes can range from cold, detached, and un-nurturing with no real boundaries to intergenerational sexual abuse with adults who sadistically control almost every behavior that the child has. And, there are plenty of variations in between.

While it is not in the scope of this book to explore all the terrible manifestations of how adults can abuse their children, it is incumbent upon clinicians treating such children to become familiar with the theories and types of neglect, abuse, and torture that children may suffer. It also is a good idea to give some attention and study to the local child protective agencies and State laws governing child welfare.

Not every case of neglect or child abuse may be interpreted by the child victim as traumatic in the sense of long term symptom formation, though the nature of the critical incident (abuse), frequency, and duration would clearly be instrumental. While there is an *objective* difference between a first time (and only time) bruising of a child from a physical strike by an adult and the same behavior repeated to varying degrees over the course of years, the single, one-time event *subjective experience* of the child *could* very well result in the formation of long term stress symptoms.

A primary key in recovery for child abuse victims is the establishment of an environment that can provide very high nurturing and very high levels of structure. "High nurture-high structure" is a broad brush way of implying a great many healthier facets of family life than the child has experienced in the time of their abuse. It does not necessarily follow that this kind of environment cannot be established in the child's home of origin. In some cases, the adult perpetrator has been forced to leave the home where the abuse occurred, and the remaining adult may have the ability to learn (or is being forced to by the Court) how to provide the needed "high nurture-high structure" for the child.

When the child is left in the home where the abuse occurred, treatment is likely to be slow going: the adult caregiver may not fully "get on board" the treatment plan, or be consistent in their giving "high nurture-high structure", and, the child is left in a home environment that holds multiple cues to their trauma.

Fortunately, there is foster care placement for abused children. Unfortunately, most funding for foster care is complex, dicey, and notoriously underfunded at local, State, and national levels. There is clearly a better chance to create the "high nurture-high structure" environment in a foster home than the home that reminds the child of their abuse.

Foster parents are very special people. They take in often much damaged children and parent them as if they were their own. While there are some foster parents with questionable motivation and caregiving out there, the majority of foster parents are good people who have been motivated by love (and many by faith) to do the work that they do, often for inadequate compensation. It is important to remember that it is not only "strange" for the abused child to go and live at someone else's home, it is equally "strange" for the foster parents and natural children.

Children who have had traumatic reactions to abuse will obviously have difficulty in trusting, accepting structure from foster parents, and likely have grave reluctance to accept nurturing gestures. This can be because of the fact of the placement in a strange new place, or it can be just a continuation of their useful and effective behavioral defenses that they used when they were in the abusive situation. The foster parents need to have well rehearsed, specific, clear communications about structure in the home, and have multiple creative means to demonstrate high nurturing in a way that the child is able to accept and use.

For many children finding themselves in foster care, their experiences of home life has included very inconsistent structure and nurturing. For example, the child whose single parent abuses substances may go long periods without either nurturing or structure. Then, when the parent decides to "clean up" for while, the parent tries to overcompensate for the lost time by "smother nurturing" and / or "drill sergeant discipline". It takes little imagination to see the behavioral problems that can develop when a child enters a home where nurture and structure are consistent.

The environment that treatment takes place in for stress disordered children needs to be one of very consistent high nurture and high structure. When a trauma happens to a child, their sense of safety is compromised; they look to their adult caregivers for demonstrations of a return to normalcy and security. High nurturing and structure does this well. It is well known that children want adults to give them limits (structure). In this sense, the structure becomes a nurturing response to the child.

Everyone needs some predictability in their lives, just as everyone needs some structure in order to go about their duties. Children as well as adults need structure in their lives in order to function comfortably. Often, children who have had very difficult histories are in special need of a higher amount of structure in order to correct negative behaviors that they have learned.

Aside from their trauma experiences, these children may have had either little structure or inconsistent structure. "Structure" covers many things: daily routine, predictability of events, assigned chores and tasks, accountability for who is in charge, how disagreements are processed, how discipline is carried out and above all, *and impeccable consistency* in all of these areas.

When children have not had enough structure, or the structure has been very inconsistent, they begin to develop multiple layers of behavioral difficulties beyond their trauma symptoms, and become unstable emotionally. Sometimes, they become "wild" in their behaviors. Other times they may become quite "parentified" taking on the role of structuring their lives and their younger siblings lives in replacement of adults.

When children spontaneously take up a stabilizing role in disorganized situations, it is a proof that human beings want structure and naturally tend to organize their lives. In any case, children who have had little structure are often dealing with significant levels of stress *in addition to their trauma history*. Even adults become stressed when their lives become unpredictable for extended periods of time. This stress will be expressed in acting out behaviors of some sort, guaranteed. Structure provides predictability, predictability lowers stress, and lower stress produces a more stable child.

Interestingly, children who have lived for some time without age normal structure will often become upset when structure is then placed upon them. These children may resent that the relative freedoms of having little structure are being removed. These children also are often quite sensitive to disruption of structure once it is established. They need to learn to accept age normative structure from caregivers, as well as appropriate flexibility in that structure.

We need to help them to trade this "freedom" for age appropriate structure as something that will offer them a payoff. While trying to replace little structure with a higher structure, we need to be sure to offer a great deal of nurturing and security. Eventually, the structure we give them will help begin to heal their old wounds, feed nurturing needs that are unmet, and provide security and comfort to them.

All Structures Change

From time to time we all change our structures (for example, as I write this, the seasonal time change has just occurred, requiring adjustments). For children with difficult histories, we need to be especially aware of each child's unique structural needs. Too much structure and the child will (rightly) rebel. Too little, and acting out begins. Often, you will know when a child needs more structure, because their behavior will tell you. It might pay off to attend closer to this when household structure is naturally disrupted, like for a holiday, or having houseguests. Compensating by giving more nurturing attention and behavioral support can make the changed structure and routine easier to sail through.

When children seem to be out of control in the home for more than a few moments (or a day), it is important to review the current structure of the household, and help the caregiver to make adjustments if needed. Caregivers are often too busy and too close to their own lives to recognize structural problem areas. The clinician can volunteer to be an in-home observer to help the caregiver get unstuck. It is a good idea to be direct in your approach to the caregiver, making specific, practical suggestions given not only verbally, but in a written list that you can leave with the caregiver.

A higher level of structure is indicated in both parent and foster parent led homes. In most average and fairly healthy homes, structure can vary from day to day and month to month (like from school year to summer time). Even this normal flux may be triggering to a stress disordered child.

In a recent situation in my work as a Behavior Specialist, a three year old girl entered into a severe, two day stress episode, because the foster parents began to take down their Christmas tree and pack away ornaments. The holiday season had been less structured than normal, and the little girl also was reminded by the packing that in her short life, she and her mother had moved many times, often in the middle of the night to avoid the landlord.

Educating Caregivers

Educating caregivers to increase their structure by communicating clearly to the child about what is going to happen next, and why, can help compensate in such situations. Understandings we adults take for granted may be quite severely misinterpreted by the PTSD child. Often, caregivers need to repeat their reassurances several times, in different ways before the child can reflect back their correct understanding.

Besides a focus on greater structure through increased and clear verbal communication, caregivers can also provide the child with visual helps such as a large calendar that is placed at the child's eye level. This then can include stickers or color codes that can be easily understood by the (non-reading) child. Knowing what events and activities are coming up can be tremendously comforting as well as structuring.

The importance of structure

Daily structure should be as routine and predictable as possible. There should be a very narrow amount of "free time" in the stress disordered child's life. Any changes of routine should be communicated verbally and on the child's calendar as soon as the alteration is known.

Caregivers should be advised to structure routine time for adults and children to be together one on one and as a whole family. Though it may sound like an oxymoron, there also needs to be time structured to have spontaneous, <u>un</u>structured fun. Such times offer the child some freedom to be silly, and options for in the moment activities. It also fosters the ability to cope and set self made boundaries in less than (highly) structured situations.

Increasing nurture may be a bit more complex and challenging for both natural parents and non-related caregivers. "Nurture" can mean many different behaviors that are expressed differently depending on the child's age or developmental level. For example, humor can be quite nurturing, but what if you care for an adolescent that has a much younger child's emotional "IQ"?

How we nurture others is largely learned through how we ourselves were nurtured. While this may be adequate if the only children we are nurturing are our own (and they are not PTSD), if we are working with a damaged child, more specific and targeted nurturing behaviors will need to be learned and practiced as well as taught to and practiced by the caregiver.

At its most basic, nurturing can be divided into two categories of our purposes: verbal and non-verbal behavioral demonstrations of care, concern, and support. Both are important to demonstrate, and one without the other is not nearly as effective. Most people tend to use either verbal or non-verbal nurturing more. Also, most of us use nurturing in a spontaneous manner; that is, we don't *plan or think* about it very much. In treating children and teens with PTSD, much more *planning and thinking* about it is in order.

Caregiving encompasses quite a multitude of verbal and non-verbal behaviors. Offering empathy when appropriate, bringing someone a cup of tea or chicken soup when they are sick with a cold point to this kind of combination of verbal and non-verbal behavioral set that communicates nurturing and care. While these may seem obvious, it may not be so obvious that such caregiving tends to drop off when the person we are caring for is healthier and more stable. It is very important to understand that PTSD children may often look more healthy and stable than they really are. Even when the child looks "OK", caregivers need to provide an increased level of caregiving behaviors as part of the child's treatment.

Affection

Affection certainly can be communicated by caregiving behaviors, but it also needs to have some specific and "clear boundary behaviors." Each child should be assessed as to their comfort level and growth potential for moving into physical and verbal affection.

Victims of physical or sexual abuse may be very cautious of physical contact of any kind, so caregivers should not automatically assume that they can hug the child, for example. Setting a rule of "ask before you touch" is a way to demonstrate both respect and by extension, affection. If the child shows severe discomfort and reluctance for "close" affection like hugs, "high fives", handshakes, or pats on the back can serve well.

In foster care situations, the question often comes up: what should the child call the foster parents? The verbal demonstration of affection of "Mom and Dad" is one not to be taken lightly. It is very fair (and healthy) for the foster parents to have a clear boundary what they are comfortable with.

Keeping in mind that many foster parents either go immediately to "call me Dad" or "call me John", I would suggest several "levels" of how the child should refer to the foster parents, with each level having a specific and therapeutic purpose (not to mention *structure.)* For the first month or two of care, the child should refer to the foster parent as "Mr. or Mrs." in front of their *surname*. This establishes a tone of respect that the child likely needs to learn and practice. It also makes a statement about how healthy relationships *develop over time.*

When the child has demonstrated consistent respect, the second level can be *negotiated*. I would suggest that the foster parent and child develop a respectful, but affectionate nick name, but it needs to be prefaced with "Mr." or "Mrs." For example, a child might call me "Mister Bill", or "Mr. K."

Later, possibilities could be derivations of "Mother" or "Father" that the child *does not call* their own parent(s): "Pop", "Mam", etc. This measure is to help the child comfortably avoid the loyalty issues that are inherent in calling someone other than your biological parent "Mom" or "Dad". It also allows the child to have a name for the caregiver that demonstrates the uniqueness of the foster parent-child relationship alongside the developed affection.

Likewise, the foster parent should demonstrate a high level of respect to the child by making sure they *first ask* the child what they prefer to be called (Robert or Bobby, for example.) Remember that a person's name is extremely personal. There have been times when a child tries to call me "Billy". While I allow "Bill", only a handful of people in my life are allowed to call me "Billy."

Humor

Humor can be very nurturing, if everyone in the home is on the "same page". One foster home I work in makes it a point to help abused and neglected children learn the difference between cruel, cutting down humor and pleasant family humor, like gentle ribbing. Children coming out of homes where part of the abuse was exposure to addicted adults, often have a hard time gauging other people's interactions with them. Addicted adults are notoriously unpredictable in their mood, affect, and interaction behaviors. Once children can "get the jokes" in the caregiving family, they tend to become much more comfortable and settled in. The private, inside jokes of a family dynamic provides an intimate and often profound connection between the foster child and foster family.

On the other side of the coin, if the child is remaining in their biological home, the clinician may need to assess the types and levels of humor that are used in the home. If the type of humor is cutting and relentlessly teasing for example, this can clearly add to the child's stress load. One can even make a case for PTSD developing just from relentless, harassing teasing of an individual. In addition, some families have a high degree of sexualized humor in their dynamic. This too is stressful for children, and should be curtailed to at least exclude the children from.

Compliments are a complex form of nurturing

The giver needs to be very aware of how a selected individual will receive the compliment effort. What may be complimentary to one person is not to another. For example, many people enjoy compliments about the way they dress. In this writer's case, I have never found pleasure in having someone tell me I "look nice". While I fully understand and accept that dressing certain ways is needed for certain situations, I don't feel that I have just received a compliment that has meaning for me (though I do say "thank you"!)

If a child is coming from a home that has given only a few genuine compliments in the child's lifetime, the child may have a difficult time believing the compliments that the clinician or foster parents give. Thoughtful and genuine complimenting is quite an art.

First, you can make a choice between complimenting a talent, a desired routine behavior, a clear effort at changing an undesired behavior, or honoring a character strength. The trick is to be sure that what you choose to compliment has a high probability of being valuable to the person you are complimenting. For example, if a child clearly values keeping their belongings in order, compliment that, instead of how well they tie their shoes.

Perhaps the least used compliments are those that address a person's character. It is curious that this is so, because in my experience, these are usually the most powerful compliments that be given. Perhaps they are given less because they indicate that the giver is intimate enough to recognize these very personal aspects of the receiver. Such a level of intimacy can be uncomfortable for the receiver, and for some givers (clinicians.) Telling someone that you can see how kind they are, or that you have discovered how courageous they have been to survive the horrible things that have happened to them can be a profoundly meaningful compliment.

The Unindulgent Favor

Being kind does not cost very much! Day to day kindness is something that many people have lived without. As a former Boy Scout Leader, who had never been a Boy Scout, one of the most impressive traditions of that program is that a Scout should "do a good turn daily". Since I was teaching this to my sons in the Scouting Program, it was incumbent upon me to model the behavior. It may sound trivial, but the practice of doing "good turns" changed my way of interacting with other people. I use the admittedly made up word "unindulgent" to indicate that some folks confuse "favors" with "indulgences". Also, a favor should be something kind you *do* for another person that does not necessarily involve a physical item. "Do me a favor and buy me that item" is not a favor, it is an indulgence.

Motivation is the key in distinguishing if a favor is a real favor. If the favor is being done to placate the other person, then it is not a favor, it's an indulgence or a bribe. If the favor is being done out of a sense of debt, as in: "I did that for you, now you have to do this for me", then there are no favors involved. The true test of nurturing favors is when the giver *chooses* to do kind favors for the receiver even when their relationship is stressed. The power of this kind of nurturing with stress disordered children should not be underestimated. For many such children, all favors in their lives have been quid pro quo.

Emotional attending

Emotional attending is a basic way we nurture others, as every clinician well understands. While clinicians make heavy use of attending behaviors early in treatment to "join with" or "develop a therapeutic alliance", it is has been my experience that in work with children who have stress disorders, there is a need for a higher level of attention given to ongoing maintenance of emotional attending. This fact needs to be shared consistently with the caregivers.

The reader will please recall my statement earlier in the book that for some reason, some people have a very difficult time accepting that some behaviors they see out of a stress disordered child are not simply oppositional, tantrums, or manipulations, but have their source in the child's trauma history. If treatment team members do not remember this, they may revert back to more familiar techniques associated with treating genuine opposition and manipulative children (which do not work with PTSD.) This is not, of course, to say that stress disordered children will not be oppositional, have tantrums, or manipulate from time to time.

Once again, "emotional attending" should not be interpreted to mean "emotional indulgence". It's just the opposite, in fact. Giving the child the freedom to express their emotions is therapeutic, especially for those children who have lived in situations where the only legitimate emotional expression allowed was by the abusive adult. In this sense, "attending" becomes literally a continual monitoring of the child's moods and affect as a tool for treatment and evaluation of treatment success.

Empathy

Offering empathy should never be seen as indulgent. Empathy is a powerful behavior of nurturing. When it is given properly, the receiver can feel that the giver really cares about them, and that what they are going through is not trivial. Clinicians need to make it a part of their effort to help the caregiver of the child to learn the ins and outs of empathy: how and when to express empathy and that empathy does not mean condoning of misbehaviors, violent behavior, or self-harm.

In my experience in working with caregivers, one of the maintenance duties I regularly perform is emotionally attending to the caregivers themselves. Working daily with a stress disordered child can be quite exhausting physically and emotionally. Since stress disorders profoundly alter a child's attachment abilities, they can be *relentless* in their defensive, challenging, and pushing away behaviors with caregivers.

Compassion fatigue in the caregiver results, and needs to be monitored by the clinician. When the ability for the caregiver to provide empathy drops, the clinician needs to make an intervention of some sort, whether a pep talk to the caregiver, or seeking out a respite time for both child and caregiver.

Eye Contact

Eye contact, as we all know, is a fundamental of emotional attending and high end communication. It is also a very intimate behavior that even clinicians some-times are uncomfortable with, so imagine how much more difficulty a child who has been abused may have with it? I have watched fellow clinicians and caregivers *demand* eye contact from a child in the most insensitive ways and situations possible.

While there are times to *direct* a child to give eye contact, those "times" need to be articulated and differentiated from other therapeutic types and purposes of eye contact. It should be recognized that such demands are likely a misjudged idea of demonstration of respect on the part of the 'demander'. In fact, the child's abuse perpetrator may have conditioned the child to *not look into the perpetrator's eyes, lest a greater amount of abuse be showered down upon the child.* The reader can clearly see the implications of how such demands could trigger a stress episode in the child.

First, there needs to be recognition between eye contact at times when the child is in a stress episode versus eye contact in day to day situations when the child is not in a stress episode. Further, in day to day situations, there needs to be a differentiation between eye contact in giving directives, and eye contact in offering nurturing. Firmly and kindly directing any child to give you eye contact prior to an important communication is a wise routine to establish. Demanding eye contact during a stress episode is another matter. This is an indication that the "helper" is totally ignorant of the source of the behavioral upset that the child is having, and needs more education on PTSD in children.

During initial work with a child, I try to build eye contact time by simply "catching" the child's eyes on mine, and, well… focusing on making my eyes *gentle*. I usually try to add a smile of encouragement to the child. By consciously focusing on this behavior in the early stages, the frequency of eye contact will increase, often dramatically.

Being an amateur magician, I often use small magic tricks as a means of capturing eye contact in a non-threatening format. Establishing the safety for the child to look into my eyes will pay off later, when they are willing to look into my eyes so that I can deliver my nurturing messages. Of course, caregivers need to learn this too, and the clinician may need to give an explicit, modeling lesson for the caregiver.

I suppose that it may be my Pastoral Counseling background, as well as my nature, that leads me to believe in the power of eye contact in helping other people. For me, for two people to really trust and touch each other at the "heart" level, eye contact must be present in such intimate work as healing.

Unconditional Positive Regard

Unconditional positive regard is a phrase that has been around for quite some time in the helping profession (how long ago did I first read Carl Rogers?) Abused and neglected children carry much "conditional" baggage in their lives. Traumatized children already feel different than their peers, and not positively so. Conditional demonstrations of caring and nurturing may be all these children have ever experienced, and all that they know how to demonstrate themselves towards others.

In direct clinical work, the abused child will classically withhold details of their difficult life, not only because of the characteristics of PTSD, but because the child has learned that if they share details of their trauma, others may reject them. Most people are very uncomfortable when they hear the raw details of a person's trauma; it's just very hard to tolerate much of. While the naïve listener may not be actually rejecting the victim, the listener's reaction (read 'rejection' of the details) can be interpreted by the victim as rejection of himself or herself. Thus, when the time comes for the victim to be finally comfortable with us to tell the details of their story, our nurturing by way of unconditional positive regard for them is likely the motivating force that allowed them to do this in the first place.

Work may need to be done in helping the caregiver understand that there is difference between unconditional positive regard and allowing the child to use their trauma history as an excuse for poor behavior. Simply taught, the caregiver always cares for the child, but does not unconditionally condone all the behaviors that the child demonstrates.

Work alongside a child for a while, and anyone will recognize how such activity can be nurturing (for both child and adult). Some of my best personal moments in counseling and time spent with my sons have been when I was 'working alongside'. I am using the word 'work' here to mean not just work, but play and adventure as well.

Shared experiences can bond people together (just look at war), but the experiences do not have to be dramatic or traumatic. In clinical practice, this can be something as simple as completing a puzzle with the child, or helping with a tough homework problem, or helping to teach how to do a household chore. Caregivers can find hundreds of ways to 'work alongside" the child, from planting the family garden to getting the campfire started to cook food on the camping trip.

Accept nurturing

Allow yourself to be the receiver of the child's efforts to nurture. Many years ago, within the first couple of years of doing Mobile Therapy, a boy of about eight that I was treating apparently noticed that I was a bit 'down.' He took a flat, amber colored glass marble that is used as a game marker out of his pocket, held it up to the sun and said: "When you look at the light through the marble, it makes you feel happy…here, it's a present for you." To say that this was a breakthrough in his treatment is an understatement; as it also was a starling and genuine gift to me that I will never forget. (In fact, I still have that glass marker, and look through it when I am feeling down!)

When we allow such expressions from the children we treat, we are not only building bonding to further treatment, or giving them practice in kind giving, we are graciously receiving appropriate support and thanks for what we do for the child. Again, caregivers may need to be instructed to watch closely for subtle gestures that the child may begin with to 'give back' to them. Like most of us, children will begin with only small efforts of care demonstration, and these could be easily missed or ignored by busy caregivers. Warm acknowledgement of the child's giving to us results in mutual nurturing that is healthy and wonderful!

11 | Helping to Break Negative Engagement Patterns

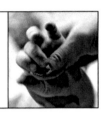

Highly and chronically stressed children tend to engage with others in a variety of negative fashions: they may present as reticent, overtly shy and regressed, or they may present as aggressive, offensive, and contrary. In some children, these presentations alternate, which may lead to the misdiagnosis of bi-polar disorder. At any rate, the stressed child has often been stuck in negative engagement patterns for a very long time, even their entire life. It becomes imperative to disrupt this pattern as a tool for healing.

Human patterning is a very strong force that is highly resilient. Altering behavioral patterns of interaction and engagement are a real challenge (as any therapist who has worked with a borderline personality knows). The negative pattern exists *because it worked.* People tend to repeat what works, and in the case of an abused child, they wisely do not want to give up old patterns for new ones, especially if they believe that they will still need the strategic, albeit negative pattern.

The younger the child, the easier the task of re-patterning can be, but it still poses a need for extensive patience and steadfast repetition on the part of the caregiver. Stress disordered children are extremely persistent in their negative engagements, and this makes it hard for caregivers to cope; caregivers need specific training on how to interrupt and respond to the child's attempts to engage negatively.

In naive terms, the child may be said to be engaging negatively "just to get attention". While this is true in the broad sense, the phrase "just to get attention" needs to be unpacked for details. Everyone needs a certain amount of attention from others; this is a basic premise for interaction. The danger of simplifying the negative engagement in this way is to allow dismissal of the underlying causes and genuine needs. When a fellow professional uses this term in a fashion as if it were a diagnostic criteria, I usually quickly follow with the question: "And so what is wrong with wanting and getting attention?"

Of course, the answer to the question is "nothing." The problem is *how* the child is seeking the attention and *how* they are habituated in engaging to get their needs met. Children who have been in chaotic households or abusive households have developed aberrant ways of engagement to get their needs met. The child who whimpers and pouts to apply guilt pressure to an inadequate parent who indeed should feel guilty and the aggressive, bossy, and loud child who uses this strategy to keep their perpetrator at bay while still demanding that their needs are met are just two variations that the reader can use to imagine still others. It is important to emphasize that the child may not negatively engage to *seek some benefit or to get a basic need met,* they may also negatively engage as a defense against further abuse.

The habituated engagement patterns, especially those that are used as defensive measures against further abuse are likely closely tied in to the allostatic process. When the child feels as if they are under threat, the reflexive chemical process boosts the automatic reactions that may have served to keep them safe in the past; in this case, aggressive and loud opposition

If the abused and stressed child enters into a foster home, they will likely continue to use their familiar patterns of engagement in order to make their needs known, or as a routine approach to the unknown quantity of an unfamiliar caregiver. In cases where the child has been exposed to many new and unfamiliar people who may have abused them, this very cautious and defensive engagement routine can be seen as quite reasonable, if not wise.

The process of altering the negative engagement patterns will be that much easier in a foster home that presumably, has a higher level of functioning, health, and positive engagement than it will be if the child continues to live in the home that they were traumatized in. Other variables in the difficulty or ease of changing the patterns are the type and extent of the child's abuse, how old the child is, and the relative intellectual abilities of the child. Generally, the longer the pattern has existed (the age of the child), the more difficult the pattern is to extinguish.

The foster caregivers must recognize that in most cases, foster children who have high levels of stress disorder symptoms are "bottomless, dry wells" of emotional and attention neediness in addition to their habituated pattern of negative engagement. So, the first and deceptively simple task is to "feed the need" that the child has before they begin to engage in their negative pattern of engagement. Deceptively simple, because this is easier said than done; the shear neediness of these children can be quite simply overwhelming. And, being highly nurturing to an aggressive child is counter-intuitive.

Careful observations by the clinician of the child in the caregiver home will yield the needed information on how the child negatively engages adults for the things the child needs, and in turn point to the particular areas of need that the child expresses most often. These "needy developmental areas" should be clarified and addressed as a supportive treatment element.

These needy areas typically surround gaps in the child's sense of safety, security, identity, ego boundary, and self image or self-esteem. If the child has experienced their trauma very early in life, there is likely a very strong element of nurturing need that requires fulfillment on a frequent basis. A fine standard is to instruct caregivers to first gain a good understanding of what the average, undamaged child's emotional, supportive, nurturing, and psychological needs are, then double or triple what is done by the adult to satisfy the average child's needs.

The next part of training the caregiver is to teach them how and when to block a child's negative engagements. A protocol can be developed that is then written down for the caregiver to refer to until they can carry it out by rote. Insistence that eye contact is given during engagement, interrupting the child if their tone is whining, regresses, aggressive, demanding or disrespectful are elements of the protocol. All of the skills that will be cited in the next chapter of this text apply to this endeavor.

The caregiver also needs to learn how to "pick their battles"; not every negative engagement tactic that the child uses needs or should be met with correction and resistance. Sometimes, the experienced and skilled caregiver can maneuver to take the wind out of the child's sails by making a quick and accurate interpretation of what the child's genuine need is, and then fulfilling it. Or, they learn that there are times to simply ignore the child's comments and behaviors.

If the child continues to have court ordered contact with biological family members who they are highly reactive to, the process of re-patterning will take longer. If the goal is for reunification, there is an ethical element to expecting or insisting that the child give up strategies and patterns that they still may need to get their needs met and to avoid abuse in the future. Children can, despite this, learn to alter their engagement style with other adults in their lives that they learn to assess as "safe".

Altering an abused child's negative interaction style is not easy work; it has to go on day after day with patient, kind, and knowledgeable adults. Not only does the alteration of the negative engagements patterns help the child heal old wounds by the repeated positive interaction, but it also is training to help the child be more successful in their here and now, as well as their future interactions.

12 Face-to-Face Gentling Countenance

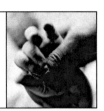

Voice tone is measured as equally important as verbal content in the Gentling approach. The easiest way to express exactly *what* basic tone to use is to point to Mister Rogers. Just one reason *Mister Roger's Neighborhood* has been such a popular and effective television program for children is that Fred understood how important it was to speak to children with kindness and gentleness, along with deep respect for their intelligence and dignity. He projected a kind of confidence, strength, and firmness that served to enhance his gentle countenance. Those who have made fun of how Mister Rogers spoke during his TV broadcasts (including all those bad imitations) have apparently never actually tried to relate to a child in this manner. It is not as simple or as easy as it first appears.

Voice tone includes much more than the actual acoustical values of a human voice. It includes volume, pace, the choice of words used, speed of the speech, and the relative mood of the person speaking. There are also characteristics that are rather tough to tie down with descriptors, such as confidence, respect, dignity, and strength. And of course, there is gentleness itself. When all of these are effectively combined in speaking to a damaged child, healing behaviors, hearts, memories, and spirits begins in earnest.

In general terms, the Gentling Approach makes use of the following combinations of voice tone:

- kind and firm
- low and slow
- soft and nurturing
- soft and empathetic
- neutral and directing

The following voice tones are actively avoided:

- loud and demanding

- sarcastic and teasing
- fast and bossy
- quiet and conspiratorial

The reader will quickly see what is being pointed to: avoid speaking in fashions that may be reminiscent of the child's experience of interactions with the perpetrators of their abuse.

Voice volume does not necessarily need to always be low, though there are important times when it should be. The gentling approach makes use of the full range of vocal volume, from barely audible whispers to really good shouts. A shout can't be gentle, you say? I would disagree. How about a shouted invitation to go fly a kite with me on a warm, breezy day? A voice cannot be both firm and gentle you say?

Firmness requires loud volume, then? I would disagree again. How about a gentle firm direction to sit down so that I can bandage your skinned knee? In later chapters that revisit treatment objectives, the reader will be cued on what vocal characteristics to use in particular situations.

The *pace* at which a person talks probably depends on two basic things: habit and their stress level. While some few people slow down their speech under stress, most of us would agree that we talk faster. Don't you hate it when someone leaves their phone number on your message service, and you have to play it five times to get the number because the person is talking too fast?

Even though I am very busy most of the time, I make sure that I give my phone number very slowly. It's is not just a practical exercise to help others get the number correctly; when I slow it down, it demonstrates a kind of respect and care for the receiver. It also helps me to (appear, at least) unstressed and in control of my day. When we present ourselves in a helping relationship as calm and having our own stress under control, this of course, engenders confidence in the person we are trying to help.

Especially with children, pace is important because they may not understand all of the words we adults use. Professional helpers also can slide into using clinical words and expressions that children (and many adults) just do not understand. And it is human nature to just nod your head, like you "get" what the other person is saying. If exercising a slower pace *conveys* calm and low stress, it also can "carry along" the person you are helping into that more relaxed place. And let's face it, a slower pace is gentle…think of a vacation in the South Pacific, lying in a hammock, living life at a snail's pace.

Another bad habit people in day to day life have is that they do not give *adequate time for a response.* Don't ask me how my day is, and then rush off without giving me time to tell you. The world pace seems to get faster and faster each day. Fast talkers tend to demand equally fast responses. Being rushed is not pleasant. The feeling can begin to tell the receiver that they are just another number, customer, widget, or problem.

Rushing others also tends to press *reactivity* out of them, not a well thought out *response*. Sometimes, *deciding* when you are a child is a tough thing to do, and adults do not always give children the time to think about their response (though we drill them over and over to 'think before you act'.) Remember that silence in therapeutic work is never really silent, there is a lot going on during that time.

Respect and dignity are a critical part of the proper voice tone for the Gentling approach. It makes use of the ideas above to convey to the receiver that they are respected and their dignity is valued. Respect and dignity serve the therapeutic agenda, because in work with children who have been traumatized by neglect or abuse, they may have experienced precious little of both. They also relate to the therapeutic agenda because as mentioned previously, it is very important to respect the child's pace in the healing process. Pushing the process of the therapeutic agenda is deeply disrespectful. Making the mistake of using behavior modification techniques at the wrong times in the treatment effort is also deeply disrespectful of the child's trauma experience.

Adults often tend to ignore using gestures of respect for children that they demand to be given to themselves. Many adults hold a double standard for the amount, quality, and duration of respect that they will offer to the child as opposed to what they expect back from the child. There is an enacted belief that children somehow deserve less respect and dignity than fellow adults. Hogwash!

Abandoning respect gestures towards children happen to a greater extent when the child is in the midst of acting out or are in a stress episode. Some adult caregivers have the terribly mistaken idea that they do not have to give respect to a child who is not currently demonstrating respect for the adult. There are even clinicians that follow this error into its inevitable conclusion, which is the cessation of any real therapeutic work with the child. Can you blame a client for not working because they do not feel respected by the helper? Essentially, if we believe that the child's behavior problems are a *behavioral health* problem, then we are obliged to keep in mind that while exhibiting difficult behaviors the child is suffering. Our exhibitions of respect at these times are possibly even more important than at other times.

It must be realized and remembered that when a child is experiencing symptoms of their mental health disorder, they may not be able to demonstrate respect. This is not to say that caregivers should just passively "take' the abuse from the child. It is to say that acceptance and understanding of the child's illness will engender compassion in the caregiver, making the unconditional respect giving easier. Helpers need to be able to hold onto themselves under the stress of the stressing child well enough to be able to make a difference.

Respect and dignity gestures mean that a very intentional and focused effort is made to protect the child's privacy not just through paperwork confidentiality, but also in actual practice. In treating physical ills in hospitals, good practice dictates that patients are given respect and dignity by staff 'draping' the patient's body. Mental health healing is no different. Making sure that the child is able to have reasonable privacy when they are in a stress episode, offering a tissue for a tearful child, or stating empathy are all tangible and valuable demonstrations of respect and dignity.

At first, the idea of consistently giving children *choices and options* does not appear to have much to do with gentleness in treatment, but stop and think for a moment about the last time you had contact with someone who "bulldozed" their way over your choices and options. It probably felt rather brutal. Again consider the neglected and abused child: they have likely had few real choices and options in their life, and none about the delivery of their abuse. For instance, the little girl who must choose either to have sex with her mother's boyfriend, or risk the boyfriend becoming enraged and beating up her mother. Forced 'choices' or two equally appalling 'options' do not qualify as genuine choice or option.

Structuring genuine choices and options to the age level of the child offers the respect and dignity that is spoken of above. The choices and options given at first need to be focused on pleasant, or at least neutral areas, such as choosing either cake or ice crème for dessert, or taking your shower before or after dinner. Having real choices for children who have been traumatized by neglect or abuse is a luxury to them that conveys gentle kindness.

Confidence, firmness, and strength are close cousins to each other, and spring out of the Gentling family tree. It is often said that it takes a strong person to be able to be gentle. Boys are often told that real strength is in avoiding the fight, and it takes a strong man who is confident in his masculinity to be able to show his painful emotions.

Girls are told that assertive confidence and firm resolve are hallmarks of a strong and successful woman. All of these are certainly true for adult caregivers, too. Confidence, firmness, and strength that the caregiver demonstrates, conveys that the helper is providing a 'safe harbor" for the child. Safe harbors are generally safe because their waters are calm and gentle.

As any clinician knows, *word choice or content choice* is a fundamental part of doing therapy. In doing therapy with children, a whole book could be written just on this topic! However, a few areas critical to work with children who suffer from

PTSD will be highlighted here. Careful word choice and content choice can actually enhance the Gentling therapeutic environment.

Perhaps the first consideration is what *not* to say. "Shop language" has no place with children. A child cannot effectively use a statement like: "You are being oppositional, and you know that the contingency is that when this occurs, a negative reinforcer will be applied." While a bit over exaggerated, the reader will get the point. Direct, simple, and brief sentences are best. "You are not doing what I told you to do. When this happens, you have to go to time out."

Once a satisfying word choice combination is discovered, it is a good idea to write it down so that it can be memorized. *Consistency* in word patterns used has some power to help the child begin to see the caregiver as stable and reliable. This helps to engender a secure, safe, and gentle environment.

Using *simple words and creative words* avoids the problem of the child having to work too hard to figure out what the helper means. This may mean paying close attention to the words the *child uses* to describe their life experience. For example, one little boy I worked with described his intrusive traumatic memories as "bad remembers". Thanks to him, I have found the term to be very useful with small children.

There are times in treatment when *correct terms* rather than euphemisms become important for the actual treatment and on those occasions that the child may reveal a crime that they have been a victim of for the first time. Helping the child to learn correct terms can add to the gentle healing effort. For example, a child who has been sexually abused may use coarse euphemisms that they have learned from the perpetrator.

Since words can be powerful triggers to PTSD victims, helping the child to learn to use the correct word may serve to moderate stress reactivity enough to be able to process a critical event. If a particular word appears to escalate a child's stress, the clinician might say something to the effect: "Can you tell me what "dick" means with a different word? Can you point to what you mean? There is another word for that part: "penis". Can we use that word instead?"

Part of the brutality of child abuse and resultant trauma symptoms is that the child will often make incorrect appropriations as to the reasons why the bad thing happened to them. *Correcting mistaken appropriations* that the child has will only be believable to the child once they have a trusted relationship with the clinician. Delivery of corrections to a child's mistaken view, for example, that they somehow invited their sexual abuse must be done with explicit empathy, and gentle tone of voice and countenance. This is a very important point, and is easily missed by clinicians who "have heard it all", and who have built up (the admittedly necessary) emotional defenses needed to constantly hear very difficult and painful material from children. Without the proper empathy expression and voice tone, just telling the child that "it was not their fault" sounds shallow and unconvincing.

Calm, high level empathy expression is another key Gentling technique. This goes way beyond the familiar "reflection of feeling" statements caregivers give in routine helping sessions. Calm, high level empathy expression is a technique specifically used when the child is in the midst of a stress episode. This behavior set for the helper can feel counter intuitive and be difficult to attain and maintain, because when another person is very upset, the helper's emotions tend to escalate as well.

This technique is basically the "what do you do?" answer to those who would ordinarily be very tempted to apply a behavior modification technique to suppress what *appears* to be a manipulation, or attention seeking behavior in the child. As mentioned before, the use of such behavior techniques will likely just escalate the child further into the stress episode, which is highly undesirable.

Though calm, high level empathy expression is quite self-descriptive, the thing to remember is that it makes use of all of the other Gentling techniques in combination during the time the child is in a stress episode. More detailed examples of this important technique will be elaborated upon in the chapter on technique use in relation to the treatment objectives.

Gentle *firmness* in pressing the child to accept responsibility for their behaviors that they did while in a stress episode is a more traditional behavior approach that is very important in the process following a stress episode. The caregiver needs to be reasonably sure that the stress episode is really over before taking this step. If the episode is not really over, the child will simply escalate again.

The worry often is that the child will "manipulate" their behavior to avoid this part of the treatment. While this is a distinct possibility, a caregiver will soon be able to spot the difference between a faked stress episode and a real one. This is not to say that a faked episode cannot lead to a real one, if the child is pressed. If this occurs, the answer (despite how counter intuitive it feels) is to go back to the protocol for intervention in a stress episode.

The clear and simple message to the child following poor behaviors in a stress episode is: while it is acceptable to feel bad, it is not acceptable to behave in destructive ways. Remember that he child may have a genuinely difficult time in remembering what they did and why they did it during the stress episode. This de-briefing and responsibility accepting process should include a detailing of the sequence of events in the episode by the caregiver, pointing out the unacceptable behaviors, and affirming the child's emotions during the event.

This process accomplishes several therapeutic things. First, the child is made accountable for their poor behavior. Secondly, they are receiving a detailed briefing of what went on, which serves to help the child to bring their reactivity process into their active consciousness. This is key to helping them to become self aware, which in turn sets them up for the educational and processing steps of treatment. The following step is to give the child the appropriate consequence for the poor behaviors. The final step is to give the child the clear and simple message that while the caregiver has a problem with the poor behavior, they still care very much for the child.

As mentioned earlier in the discussion on word choice and content, as well as voice tone, what we say and how we say it is important in this approach. One technique that I have used for years, and did not even realize I was "using a technique" until a colleague brought it to my attention is that of *becoming the child's age*. The best way to describe how to begin to do this is to simply imagine yourself at the child's age.

Or, another way of describing this might be: letting the *child in you* come forward to engage the child, while the adult in you does the directing and analysis. The effect this has might be called "extra strength empathy" paired with the ability to "play". Sadly, many adults have forgotten how to play, or never really learned how to play as children.

Once again, to cite Mr. Rogers, Fred demonstrated this idea very well during his television show, most vividly when he entered into the "Land of Make Believe". Close examination of this segment of the show will reveal that there were a great many serious real life and deep topics spoken about between the characters.

Getting to this "magical place" involves all of the techniques mentioned thus far, with the addition of altering your mindset to that of a child. Meeting your client "where they are at" means willingness to get down on the floor, willingness to play dress up, be silly, and engage in make-believe. It is often said that "play is the work of children". I would suggest extending that idea to include that play is also *the language* of children. Developing a playful interaction style with the child certainly does not mean that important therapeutic work is not going on. In fact, speaking any other language than the child's may be quite limited in efficacy.

It does take practice for most adults to use this technique effectively, and at first it may feel phony or wooden. The child's response to your efforts will tell you if you are on track or not. Initially, it is best to allow the child to totally direct the (appropriate) play.

You will be able to tell when the child desires for you to lead, because *they will offer it to you*. Once you are given this gift, savor it as a sign of the child's trust in you. Be sure not to 'hog' the leadership, handing it back frequently to the child. Once you "get" this technique, it may quickly become a favorite, because it not only quickens the pace of treatment, but is actually pleasurable to engage in. And, of course, the play will tell you quite accurately what is on the child's mind. Some may doubt that a child will accept and trust an adult not just behaving like but having the countenance of a child, but in my experience, the child does not miss a beat, so to speak, when I begin to play with them.

If the child has been a victim of a sexual perpetrator, there is some risk in using this technique, as the perpetrator may have used play engagement in their crime. The child's response (or more likely, *reaction*) will let you know if this is a problem. Even if the perpetrator used play as an enticement, this does not mean that you cannot use play in your work with the child. In fact, by moving slowly and demonstrating safety in your play (as in making sure that other adults are around, and the location of the play is open, with escape routes) the effort becomes one of helping the child to begin to reclaim their right to appropriate play, and to begin to play normally again.

If you can successfully become the child's age, the impact on the treatment process can be profound. Such time spent in play advances the bonding and therapeutic alliance process at a much quicker rate than simply *watching* the child play (or just "consulting" with the caregiver!). A secondary benefit is that by placing yourself at the child's age, you begin to learn the child's language.

By this, I mean the *meta-messages,* or their total communication that includes the content, underlying emotion, body language, unconscious expressions of life experience, and unique interpretations of their world. In this sense, the child's play becomes a very intimate expression of their life, and as such, should be given all due respect. I always thank the child for playing with me when the playtime is over.

While allowing the child to direct the play and take the lead in the play, this does not mean that it should not be structured. Consideration and planning needs to be a strong element in *play structuring* during therapeutic sessions. Structuring play entails setting limits and boundaries like how long the play will last, type of play options offered, where the play will (or will not) occur, and the allowable intensity level.

It also entails making corrections of *mistaken attributions* that the child may have. By this, I mean that the child may begin to re-enact their experiences with action figures, for example, and demonstrate some of their mistaken notions about how healthy people should or do interact. Following a brief time period of the child demonstrating their stress areas with the toys, I begin to correct mistaken attributions by using *my* action figure in a positive and healthy fashion.

Though I do have a set of toys that I have in my bag, I only use these rarely, preferring to use the child's own toys when possible. My toy mainstays are what I call my "happy family" dolls, some action figures that includes some superheroes, and bunch of small picture cards of human faces in different expressive moods. I also have some outdoor toys like balls and Frisbees as well as a large box of beads and beading materials that I use when I am working with children who may be a bit too old to feel that they can play comfortably with dolls and action figures. Of course, this best applies if the clinician goes into the child's home to do work, but a child could be invited to bring toys to an office setting.

Once again, by looking closely at the meta-messages, such as toy choice, tone of play, content of play, etc, much information about the child's mood, what history issues are on their mind, and stress levels can be gained. The clinician's engagement in play can offer counter meta-messages to the child that can serve to correct mistaken attributions, and to guide the child towards healing.

13 | The Encopresis and Enuresis Problem

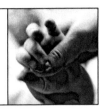

Encopresis and enuresis is almost synonymous with stress disorders in abused young children. In fact, I cannot recall a stress disordered child under the age of ten who I have treated that has not had one or both of these difficulties. Though I have not done the research on my case history, it seems as if encopresis has been much more prevalent in boys than girls. In addition to simple encopresis signs, there have been a very high number of these cases that also involve the child smearing or otherwise manipulating feces. Both problems, of course, become a sharp focus of concern and frustration for the child's caregivers.

Various theories attempt to explain why abused children develop enuresis or encopresis (in this case, defined as development following known history of adequate toilet learning). Certainly anger and rage very well could play a part, as could the idea that sexually abused children use the behaviors as a means of keeping perpetrator from repeating abuse. Intrusive dreams and nightmares about the abuse may stimulate fear responses that result in wetting or soiling. Once the pattern has begun, the bowel may get into a withholding habit that reinforces the original development of encopresis. In observing at least one eight year old male child who was in the process of playing with and smearing his feces in his bedroom, I was fascinated to observe what appeared to me to be a child in a dissociated state of consciousness. In all likelihood, the explanation might be some combination of all of these.

Whatever the source, it remains a very difficult problem for caregivers and the child. It takes little imagination of how the caregivers will approach the problem, and how these kinds of approaches serve to reinforce the problem. Thus, the caregivers need as much treatment as the child does to make it through what will be an ongoing problem. It is not unusual for the enuresis and encopresis to become *the central behavioral issue* regarding the child in the caregiving household; it can in fact become the central issue in the household, period. It is important that the clinician work hard to help the family view of the problem change, to normalize the problem as much as possible, to change focus from the child's difficult behaviors to the child's strengths, and to help the caregivers in practical ways to cope with the reality of the problem.

Caregivers need to be directed to have the child examined by a physician for any medical sources of the problem. It is critical for the physician to have foreknowledge that the child is a victim of abuse and has PTSD; this is especially true if sexual abuse is known or even suspected. In all of the PTSD cases that I have served that have had encopresis or enuresis, there never has been one that has had an identifiable physical cause. Once medically cleared, the clinician needs to work first at calming down and educating the caregiver concerning PTSD in children. It is very difficult for most adults to accept that a child who is old enough and has proven that they know how to use a toilet does not do so all of the time. It is very hard for many adults not to personalize the problem as the child being directly defiant and vengeful toward the adult. While this pattern of behavior may have had its source in such rage towards *someone*, it may not be the current caregiver.

Caregivers need to hear that the problem will likely not be solved by next weekend; in fact, it may take many months to achieve forward progress. This needs to be followed quickly by giving some very practical advice to the caregivers concerning keeping the child clean and the mitigation of damage to beds, walls, etc, establishment of a routine intervention plan with the child in response to the wetting or soiling, and emphasis on normalizing the problem and recognizing the child's strengths.

Please turn to Appendix B for a handout you can give to caregivers to deal with the practical concerns of Enuresis.

Educating Caregivers

Get all caregivers onboard, including foster parents, parents, teachers, child protection workers, and judges. The simplicity of the challenge to getting all involved caregivers on board is deceptive. As mentioned earlier, some people have a very difficult time in accepting the Gentling paradigm and understanding the subtleties of how PTSD works in children who have been victims of interpersonal trauma. Despite a culture that has widely embraced the basics of psychology, such as the concept of one's history affecting one's present, there is a large population that finds it hard to make the connection between a ten-year-old girl's severe opposition to her teacher and the fact that she was sexually violated at age three by her mother's paramour.

Each discipline, though all focused on helping the child, has their own perspective and closely held beliefs about the problems that the child has. Not only does each profession have a bias, but each individual also has a bias set, depending on his or her own particular upbringing and history. While the average person has understanding of how traumatic abuse is hurtful to a child, and are cognizant that this hurt will have some behavioral effects in the child, they will not have the more esoteric understandings of the clinician specializing in Gentling. The job is to get this motley crew of child caregivers on a single page of understanding, first of the child, and then of the signs and symptoms the child is suffering, and then the Gentling approach to treating the child.

Team approaches to treatment have distinct advantages: sharing the treatment load, access to specific expertise, and mutual supervision. But team approaches also have disadvantages: erroneous communication risks, coordination of services, disagreement about how treatment should proceed, what exact treatment approaches should be used, and the "too many cooks" effect. In many locations, there may be many professionals involved in a case for one small child.

Outpatient therapists, Mobile Therapists, Behavior Specialists, various case managers, child protection workers, lawyers, foster parents, natural parents, and police officers may all converge on a case. The team, while guided by the philosophy of "the child's best interest", may not always agree on what that exactly means. Primary to the progress of the child is that all team members accept and have a good understanding of PTSD in abused children. Many myths concerning trauma and children may need to be dispelled, that young children will 'forget quickly', or that all the child has to do is to 'keep busy' to avoid symptoms, to name just two.

Any clinician who has worked with abused children and the public service that is assigned to intervene and protect them has felt the tension between treatment and the legal system. Child protective agencies do try hard to attend both the legal requirements of needed evidence and testimony and sensitivity to the child's emotional needs, but due to this exact reason, may bobble the case ball. There is not a child protective worker with even one year of seasoning that cannot relate how they and their agency "get it from all sides" while working cases: they are pressed by the legal system to get the child to speak clearly and give painful details quickly, and pressed by counselors and therapists to be patient with the child.

The Gentling clinician understands that it may take some time for the child to begin to verbalize the fuller details of their abuse, but the court system often expects the child to be able to detail any criminal abuse that they have experienced quickly, in order to make a determination of custody, the need to remove the child from the home, or to begin legal charges against a perpetrator. The obvious problem, of course, is that the way traditional jurisprudence works is quite awkward when it comes to dealing with PTSD in children. Courts work on clear evidences and accurate, articulate witness testimony. Children with PTSD as a result of often years of interpersonal abuse rarely have either, especially if the abuse is of the more clandestine variety, like emotional and sexual abuse.

As an advocate of the child's mental health and daily functioning, clinicians find themselves in the unenviable position of educating fellow professionals in the other services. It is no surprise, of course, that all of the professionals are very busy people that do not have an hour or two to sit down and get the lecture on the nature of PTSD in abused children. One motivation for my writing this book was to be able to make the information much more accessible to judges, lawyers, child protection workers, and police officers. But aside from the hope that all of those professionals will read a copy of this book, clinicians can educate fellow professionals by carefully making use of the time they have with them.

By being careful to use correct clinical language when referring to PTSD signs and symptoms, we can accomplish two things: keep the child and their PTSD behaviors before the other professional, and perhaps press the other professional to ask for clarification about what we say. That clarification is the educational opportunity. Sometimes that need for clarification is clear, like when the fellow professional asks you to explain, but sometimes it is just a quizzical look accompanied by a pause. Don't be shy. Fill the pause with education!

Changing systems is a very hard and frustrating task. The field of child protection is just like any other; it has traditional views that are traditional with a capitol "T". These ideas and philosophies are often very entrenched and tenaciously held on to. The family preservation bias is exemplary of this kind of ensconced thinking. There are countless cases that I have worked on where although the court has stated that the child will never return to the care of the (abusive, perpetrating, unprotecting, severely triggering) parent, weekly visitations will continue. *This, despite the fact that all treating professionals on the case may feel that such visits are harming the child's ability to heal and grow.* Strong practice trends in professional fields, like family preservation, born somewhere in the early 1970s, are difficult to moderate once they are held as cover-all fundamentals.

If a clinician gets subpoenaed to testify in court regarding a child with PTSD as a result of interpersonal trauma, they have a unique opportunity to not only do their duty in testimony, but to use the platform to educate everyone involved on the nature of PTSD in victimized children. Once again, by carefully using clinically accurate (but not overly technical) language in giving testimony, education can be imparted. Below is a brief vignette:

> **Lawyer:** "So, the problem is that Janie has tantrums. Don't all children have tantrums?"
>
> **Clinician:** "Janie's upsets are different from other children's 'tantrums'. A tantrum is a way for a child to try to manipulate an adult. Tantrums have a certain kind of intensity, duration, and quality. Janie has 'stress episodes' that have a much longer duration, frequency, and intensity. Her stress episodes occur only when she had been triggered by something in her environment that reminds her of her trauma."
>
> **Lawyer:** "So, I'm still trying to understand: her tantrums last longer than most children?"
>
> **Clinician:** "Her stress episodes may last longer than a tantrum, but there are other behaviors in the stress episode that indicate that it is not a simple tantrum, such when Janie dissociates during the stress episode."

It is important for the clinician who has never testified in court concerning an abuse/PTSD case to understand their role as a witness. "Fact witnessing' is different than being an 'expert witness'. Essentially, a fact witness is just that, witnessing to facts that the clinician has experienced directly with the child, and, by their skill expertise, testifies to in court. An expert witness on the other hand, while perhaps answering many of the same questions about the disorder and common behaviors around the disorder, is being *paid* by either the defense or prosecution for their expertise. As a fact witness, the clinician is testifying to the child's condition and treatment, and is likely being paid for their services by some third party, usually a therapy service agency.

Foster parent education should be a bit easier to accomplish than biological parent training, because the foster parent is a paraprofessional being paid by some agency or the State to care for the child. Their years of experience and kind hearts can be an asset to the teaching effort. Yet, there are even some foster parents who have a very difficult time in accepting the underpinnings of PTSD understanding and Gentling approach. A key to helping people who have difficulty in this area is to give repeated teachings in various ways to help them understand and get on board the effort. Below is a brief vignette:

Foster Parent: "He just disrespects me when he gets like that. I don't tolerate disrespect from any child, not even my own!"

Clinician: "Right, I don't think you should tolerate disrespect either. Nathan must be held responsible for what he says and does in a stress episode. But let's remember that when Nathan is in a stress episode, making demands of him won't work. It works better to just help him stay safe, and talk to him gently then. After the stress episode, then you can deal with the disrespect, giving him a consequence."

Foster Parent: "I don't know if I believe that stuff about him being in a stress episode. I think he is just being a brat, and hateful."

Clinician: "Yeah, it sure is hard to hear a child talk that way to me, too. But did you notice if his eyes got glassy, and his affect went flat when he was yelling at you? Did you notice if he used that growling voice he uses when he visits his mother and is enraged?"

Foster Parent: "Yes, I guess he did all of those. It just seems like he is doing it to me just to get me mad, because he has been told 'no' about something."

Clinician: "Well, your telling him 'no' might very well be what set off that stress episode. Remember how we talked about how Nathan's mother, when she was drunk, let him do anything and everything, and when she would get sober, she would not let him do anything. He might be reacting to your 'no' as if it was his mother saying 'no' to him."

Once again, foster parents are very special people, even heroic people! But they still are human, and get frustrated and tired when children in their care who have PTSD are triggered daily, sometimes multiple times. It is hard not to take a PTSD child's stress episode behaviors personally; to remember that the behaviors are related to the child's history.

Educating biological family members is a more complex challenge. Here, the difficulty is not only presenting the information in a manner that is understandable to the family members, but this is the family context where the abuse either took place, or the child was not adequately protected. In addition, there is the overall family dynamic to contend with, along with the cognitive biases of the individual family members.

14 Stressed Self-Harm Management: Teaching Self-Comforting

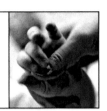

A goodly number of traumatized, abused children engage in self-harm behaviors. These behaviors may range from an extraordinary level of risk taking in play with multiple "accidental injuries" to actual direct self-harm such as biting themselves, punching themselves, or pulling out their own hair. The question becomes: why would someone hurt themselves so, when they have been hurt so badly by others? There are several possibilities that could be producing the behavior, either alone or in combination.

Anger, if not rage, would be the first suspect for such behaviors. That anger would be a reaction to abuse (especially by a loved one) that could lead to violent behavior. A child, of course, has very limited ways in which to enact their anger or seek revenge on an adult who has perpetrated abuse upon them. Not only is the adult physically bigger and stronger, the adult also likely has a strong psychological control over the child. Thus limited in emotional expression, the child may turn their rage on the most convenient target, themselves. Though rage behaviors such as violent behavior may "slide downhill" from one sibling to another, sibling on sibling violence in an abusive home may be a result of learning rather than a transference effect.

The self-harming traumatized child has lost much through the endurance of their traumas, including a loss of healthy ego identity. Remember that one effect of interpersonal trauma is that the victim loses a sense of their own ego boundary; if another person can violate their body so easily, what boundary is there? Such a loss (read: theft) of identity surely induces rage. Thus, with personal ego integrity so damaged, (read: I am not valued, I am worthless) self-harm may become an expression of this sentiment, even if it is a non sequitur.

Another possibility is that the child has used self-harm behaviors in the past because they learned these from their family of origin. It is not a stretch to conclude that if a child witnesses a suicidal gesture by others in their family that gain increased attention, sympathy, and brief cessations of abuse, the child may incorporate these into their behavior style.

Self-harm behaviors may have developed as a manipulative tool quite apart from direct observation by the child of other family members. The classic ruse of "I'll hold my breath 'till it die!" routine, if it is effectively used by the child with an adult, undoubtedly leads to negatively reinforcing such behavior. Basically, the child is counting on the adult perpetrator (or perhaps the adult who is not perpetrating, but should be protecting) to be distracted by the child's self-harm behavior and break off another round of abuse. Once this behavior is generalized, the child will continue to use it when they are under stress even when it is no longer really necessary to avoid abuse. (like in foster care).

Lastly, the trauma effects of detachment and numbing may come into play in self-harm. Having literally watched countless PTSD children injure themselves in foolish risk taking behaviors (jumping off the top step of a staircase, jumping bikes over barbed wire fences, etc.) and apparently feeling no pain, numbing and self-harm seem to present side by side. Intentional self-harm behaviors such as biting themselves, punching themselves, or head banging might be best compared to the phenomenon of "cutting" in older children (teens) and some adults. "Cutters" often state they cut because they feel numb, and want to be able to feel *something,* even if it is pain. The act of cutting is also often described in ritual, comforting, and "relief" terms.

For children traumatized by abuse, self-harm may act as means of control from becoming totally numb; "going over the edge", so to speak, and not coming back to a feeling world. The reader will realize that self-harm behaviors in PTSD children may be complex, and should not jump to a hasty conclusion about the origin (and subsequent simplistic interventions) of the behavior.

It is axiomatic that caring human being's first impulse when they see someone attempting to hurt themselves is to intervene physically. While this measure does at times need to be performed, as in the case if imminent risk of permanent damage or death, generally speaking, physical intervention with a PTSD child for any reason, including self-harm behavior is not advisable, due to the almost one hundred percent guarantee that it will just escalate their stress reaction / stress episode. Some adults find it very hard, and feel compelled to physically restrain the child, believing not to do so is irresponsible. While this is very true in cases of imminent permanent damage or death, in most cases, self-harm behaviors such as head banging, self hitting, hair pulling, biting, or breath holding do not rise to this level of need for restraint

There are studies that indicate that physical restraint in self-harm cases is not productive in ending future repetitions of self-harm. In my opinion, neither is raising your voice, demanding, or threatening consequences or forced trips to the local psychiatric hospital. So what to do? You cannot, of course, just stand by and allow a child to self-harm. You *can* attempt to ignore the *threat*, or *mild gestures* of self-harm in an effort to extinguish these behaviors. Fortunately, there are effective techniques you can use to intervene in more serious self-harm behaviors.

The first step, which should become a routine first step, is to become sensitive to the child's level of stress. Most of the time, a child will begin to self-harm only when they are highly stressed. Ideally, intervention should occur before these stress emotions get too intense, thus avoiding the self-harm behavior completely.

It is a good idea to closely observe and note the child's behavioral signs before they begin to self-harm. If you watch closely enough, you will discover a set of signs (particular to the child) that likely present each time prior to a self-harm episode. Once a child is to the point of actually doing self-harm, the described approach will likely be less effective, so it is *very important to learn the child's early, subtle signs of stress.*

Once indication of self-harm has been noted, and even when self-harm activity has begun, verbally recognize and name (to the child) the emotion you are seeing. Then, you can do a number of things, such as talk about the feelings, offer a different means to express the feelings (such as make a picture of the feeling), or help the child to refocus on something else, such as a preferred activity, or a known self-comforting behavior. It is also appropriate to invite the child to have a hug, but if they are already deeply engaged in the self-harm behavior, they will likely not take you up on this. Remember to present yourself in your voice tone, words, and countenance in a *gentling* fashion.

While it is sometimes necessary for a child to accept directives without choice, and there may come a point in this particular process to use firm directives, this is not the first option to use in self-harm situations with stressed children. The point is to continue to gently offer positive choices of different behaviors that the child could use to cope with their current emotions and self-harm behavior.

If the stress and threatened self-harm is a reaction to a directive you gave, you might want to back off a bit, and if possible, give the child a positive choice. For example, if the child begins to self-harm after a directive to take a bath, you might first recognize their emotion and reason ("I can see you are very angry at having to take a bath right now, and you might even be scared to use the bathtub"), then offer a choice ("Maybe you would like to choose if you have your bath now, or after dinner.")

If the child begins to engage in self-harm (head banging, for example), you can intervene by placing your hand, or better yet, a pillow or stuffed animal between the child's head and the wall/floor. Be sure to approach slowly, carefully, and in a non-threatening way. Ask *permission* to approach. If denied, begin to negotiate just how close is tolerable for the child. Get down on the floor with the child, don't stand over them.

So, if making demands for the behavior to stop, or trying to convince the child with logic to stop does not work, what exactly do you *say* during the intervention process? When a child engages in self-harm, I use a very gentle and nurturing voice tone and countenance, telling them that I can see how much pain they are in, and do not want to see them hurting themselves, I ask them directly to stop hurting themselves, and to take care of themselves. I may also talk about how frightening it must be to feel the way they are feeling. I then add suggestions on how they might replace their self-harm behavior with something that is better.

Keep repeating words to this effect! The child may try to remove the stuffed animal towel, or your hand, or move away from you, but be persistent in staying relatively close and putting the cushion back. You can do the same thing when a child is trying to scratch, slap, or hit themselves. You may want to get a special stuffed animal just for this purpose, and be sure to name it.

You can also ask *permission to touch* the child. Be specific in what kind of touch you intend. I find that *asking permission* to put my hand on their back is usually (if not eventually) rewarded with consent. Your touch, of course, should be nurturing and gentle. Focus your attention and the intangible "energy" of healing on the physical contact of gently rubbing the child's back, while continuing to use gentle and nurturing verbalizations.

You can also encourage the child to hug or cuddle (not hit) the stuffed animal as an alternative to their behavior. Eventually, as the child begins to settle from the gentling process, an invitation to a hug is appropriate. The idea, of course, is to teach the child a more positive way to express their emotions and needs.

Once again, knowledge of the child's abuse history is in order: such approaches as the one above may intensify the stress reactivity if the perpetrator has used similar behaviors to engage the child in abusive situations. This does not mean that the approach cannot be used with a child who has been sexually abused by a coercive perpetrator, it just means that there needs to be a high level of trust development with the child, and the process will need to go slower and with more caution than with children suffering from other kinds of abuse trauma.

It is very important to pay attention to and manage your *own emotions* during this process. If you are expressing negative emotion or highly agitated/anxious emotion, *it will make the situation worse.* You may even find yourself having a strong urge to physically restrain the child, *but don't do it, it will make the situation worse.* This urge becomes overpowering in cases where the child is say, biting themselves on the arm, and you can clearly see their teeth sunk into their arm.

In most cases, if you approach a child with the incorrect emotional expression (negative, demanding, hostile, angry), or physical posture (standing above, reaching down), they will lash out at *you* when you approach. If the child begins to lash out at you (even when you are using the correct approach), *simply move away*. Again, many adults feel an *overwhelming urge* to restrain the child at this point, but if this is done, it is a grave error that will result in escalation of intensity and frequency of the undesired behaviors.

In some ways, the fact that the child changed their focus from self-harm to lashing out at you is positive: at least they have stopped harming themselves. But on the other hand, there is a secondary problem: the child now may perceive you as a clear and dangerous threat, or even as their perpetrator. It does not take many repetitions of this sequence before you will stick in the child's mind as someone to be very wary of. This, of course, does not advance healing.

Making interventions with children who are actively involved in self-harm (or other harm) behaviors is stressful to the helper. Self-awareness of your emotional state, expression, and behaviors needs to be a continual process in these situations. If you can gain hold of your stress and tone it down, do so. If this is not possible, put considerable proximity between yourself and the child, keeping visual contact, and get backup as quickly as possible.

Even if you are doing the technique correctly, the child may calm for a short period, and then begin their self-harm behavior again. If this happens, move in with the stuffed animal and nurturing words once again. Repeat this process until the child accepts the stuffed animal without your holding it there, and calms down. Note that you may be repeating this *many* times before the child begins to accept a new way of dealing with their emotions.

This repeating effect may be a result of the stress related body chemicals re-triggering reactivity in what might be called recursive cycles. Such recursive effects will vary from episode to episode, and from child to child, and may be related to how many critical incidents have occurred to the child over a certain length of time. They may also be exacerbated by multiple repetitions of the behavior and ineffective or actual damaging approaches to intervening in them.

The question is often asked: What if the child is using self injury as a manipulative tool to avoid a non-preferred activity? Well, the child may do this to manipulate some of the time, but it will likely look different in the detail and intensity if it is studied closely. And remember, what may start out as a manipulation, can "tip over" into a genuine stress episode. In any case, you must deal with the self-harm behavior *before* addressing the manipulative behavior.

Once the child calms down, it is important to return directly back to the directive to do the non-preferred activity. Be aware that this may produce yet another round of self-harm behavior, but you must repeat the intervention *exactly* as before. It may take *many repetitions* for the child to understand that using self-harm gestures as a manipulation will no longer work.

Self-harm behaviors may be dysfunctional attempts at self-comforting, or gaining someone to provide comforting. Sometimes, a child who has been abused through emotional and physical neglect seems like (and indeed is) a "bottomless pit" of comforting neediness. Thus viewed, the need for comforting should be fed, and aggressive approaches to self-harm behaviors dropped as strategies that are doomed to fail.

Traumatized, abused children, often have never learned, use aberrant forms, or have abandoned *self comforting*. This is an important skill for them to either learn or begin to reuse, because it relates directly to their ability to self regulate their own emotions and behavior. Though a child may lean towards either a blunting of emotion (numbing and detachment) or towards physical and emotional agitation (allostatic load), they will likely have a combination of the two some degree. While at first the two symptom clusters appear to be paradoxical, they essentially are a failure to engage in self-comforting behaviors.

Of course, delivering high amounts of nurturing demonstrates to the child that they are valuable and cared for, and feeds their deep need for such demonstrations, but it does not necessarily translate into the child becoming more *self-comforting*. Towards this objective, I make a point of consistently drawing the child's attention to how well they are caring for themselves in their daily hygiene, for example. I also suggest that caregivers begin to watch the child carefully to try and ascertain if the child has any self -care behaviors that can be strengthened into more specifically self-comforting behaviors. For example, if a girl seems to give special attention to her hair, she might be encouraged to spend longer periods of time in brushing her hair, perhaps at bedtime, or when she appears to be becoming agitated to see if this is (self) comforting to her.

I also routinely speak directly about how a person "takes care of themselves". These talks range from how to be appropriately cautious around strangers or avoiding germs to literally giving yourself a hug when you need it. It is very appropriate to self-reveal how you self comfort (assuming it is healthy and appropriate!) As mentioned in a previous chapter, some children, especially those who have been sexually abused, may engage in sexual self-stimulation as a pseudo-comforting strategy.

In some sexually abused children, the self-stimulation becomes excessive and compulsive at certain times, and thus does not provide genuine self-comforting effects. Such excessive self-stimulation can also cause very real physical damages from simple irritations to bladder infections. Once again, the behavior itself may not be an inherently bad choice, but the location and compulsive frequency the child chooses to engage in may need challenging.

15 When the Child Begins to Share History

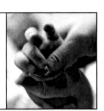

Traumatic experience negatively impacts memory. Much was made a couple of decades ago about "repressed memory"; it quickly became clear that there were many misguided if not unscrupulous clinicians who beefed up their practice by helping "victims" "recover" lost memories of abuse. This is a time in treatment of PTSD that most honorable clinicians would like to forget, but reminders perhaps serve well to guard against such repeat errors.

While some bad memories do get placed in a far distant corner of memory, they are not nearly as numerous or "repressed" as many have made a sizeable income producing out of whole cloth. Memory, for many people (even clinicians) is very tricky territory, filled with mystery and myth, half-truths and simplistic explanations. Memory is a basic psychological process that, by its nature, is always attached to subjective experience, even when it involves someone else's memory. It can be ephemeral or enduring, easily confused with dreams, and has the potential to be fragile and self-embellished, if not outright manipulated by others. A wise clinician approaches memory with the utmost care for these possible blind trails, caution concerning its objectivity, and gentleness surrounding its attached pain.

I would contend, based solely on clinical anecdotal evidence, that no one really "forgets" his or her abuse trauma. Rather, the common response appears to be for individuals, in varying degrees, to try to "put the event behind them" in order to go on with the daily tasks of living. Trying to live daily with such horrible memory "up front" may be too painful and negatively impact daily functioning far too much to be tolerable. In fact, this strategy for the individual may be a healing process. There is some evidence that a rush and press for the individual to "process" their abuse incidents is more harmful than healing. In fact, the victim's apparent refusal to confront the memories may be a functional healing tool in itself. Thus, once again, the Gentling approach does not press or rush victims to detail their trauma.

In addition to the need for a traumatized child to place traumatic memories on the "back burner" in order to function, the nature of how memory works while a trauma is occurring is important to understand. Countless psychological experiments on the nature of memory in relationship to victims and witnesses to crimes shows that there is some variability in accuracy from person to person depending on the person, the crime, the level of violence, and the age of the victim. There are likely *many* more variables that impact the memory of someone who is experiencing interpersonal trauma, including intelligence level, culture, and even time of day that the assault took place. The bottom line is that trauma places alterations and limitations on an individual's accuracy for facts.

While accuracy suffers, this suffering points to the problems of "truth". Accuracy and truth are two separate issues. Abuse can surely be "true" without an accurate accounting of details. Much research shows that while child witnesses are more or less as accurate as adult witnesses, and they generally do not falsely report abuse, they have the potential to be fairly easily led into giving details of abuse that never occurred.

Most children are socialized to either try hard please adults, or to work hard at not being caught without the proper answer that an adult expects. As a result, when adults question children, the average child will often confabulate to some degree to satisfy the relief of this pressure. In addition, younger children generally have a harder time in relating the correct sequence of facts when relating a memory. Children who have been traumatized by interpersonal violence have these tendencies magnified many times.

This is not to say, of course, that a child's statements of abuse are to be disregarded in light of the problems with trauma and memory. It simply means that the wise clinician has done their homework and has an operational understanding of what weight to give the memories that are presented in treatment, and how to avoid altering those memories in any way. Far too often, clinicians become entrapped by a "target fascination" or voyeuristic self-indulgence concerning the sordid details of the victim's abuse. Taken to extremes, this is likely the source for the "recovered memories" debacle; pressing victims to remember usually produces some very dramatic results that, when leaked into the public realm, can produce quite a community buzz (and no doubt ego boost) surrounding the name of the clinician who "specializes" in recovering memories of "victims of devil worship," for example.

I addition, there are still clinicians (despite training) who have grave difficulty in believing a child's account of events in general, let alone concerning abuse. On the other hand, there are clinicians so enamored by their own self-image as superhero to children that they take what children relate at face value. Such a bias naturally negatively influences progress in treatment. Both extremes, that a child never tells mistruths about abuse, and that children cannot be trusted to recognize fact from fantasy are both patently false.

I cannot resist telling a personal story to exemplify this point. Years ago, when my first son was in preschool, I asked him on the way home what he had done that day in school. He stated that he and the other children followed the directions of the teacher to "chop up a snake" that they had found in the play yard and "throw it over the fence". This was all allegedly done as the children danced around and sang a song.

As a young clinician (or perhaps more as a parent) who was reading in the news of horrible situations in other preschools across the nation where children were being sexually abused, my concern grew as I questioned my son. It seemed at each questioning, his detailing of the events took on a more ominous tone. Of course, as the reader has guessed, the next day yielded an explanation from the teacher of the children playing a spontaneous pretend game where a jump rope became a "snake", with the boys valiantly "chopping up the snake" and tossing it over the play yard fence. My three year old son did not lie to me, and his memory of the event was quite accurate. He just left out a few details!

Placing the clinical field's own bad memories aside, (in order to continue functioning!), there are several simple, gentle rules to keep in mind when working with memory material while treating child victims of traumatic interpersonal abuse.

Rules for working with memory material of child victims

1. The details of abuse memory are only important if they serve to either protect the child from further abuse (as in the clinician being a mandated reporter), or the *child* is using the details to work through *their* abuse. The details themselves have no magical power to help the child progress. While some research shows that some people benefit from "detailing" their specific abuse episodes, there by no means is agreement that this is a modality suited to all victims healing styles. Helping a child to understand that *some people* feel better after detailing is different than *insisting upon such detailing*.

2. Mistaken attributions associated with the memory of details are far more important to treatment than the detail itself. Often, details of the abuse are not what is "holding" the erroneous attribution; rather, the context of the abuse is. Correct mistaken attributions!

3. The victim owns their memories. It's their right to share or not to share memories at the pace that they desire and can manage. These memories are intensely private, likely embarrassing to some degree, and genuinely

painful. There is a huge difference between encouraging exploration of a memory once it is brought up and relentless pressing for details. To oversimplify and call the child "resistant to therapy" is both absurd and a sign of an over-inflated clinician's ego. Continuous and repeated pressing for details and recounting is abusive, damaging, driving symptoms deeper, and is unethical!

4. Traumatic memory, by nature, is often fuzzy. When under assault, a victims' basic task is survival, not accurate recording of details. It is likely that a rush of body chemicals are activating survival strategies, putting memory on the back burner. As such, any recounting is likely have at least parts that are quite "fuzzy". There will be parts of the memory that are quite literally gone, as in, "never even recorded to memory." What details that are intact may tend to change order sequence, or shift in emotional weight with different recounting. In children, this may lead some adults to misunderstand what is going on, and begin to accuse the child of lying. Such accusations only serve to teach the child to never speak about their abuse. Just accept fuzzy memory as a fact, and that pressing for clarity may not only be futile, but damage the treatment potential further.

5. Traumatic memory, by nature, is often disconnected. What details that are intact may tend to change order sequence, or shift in emotional weight with different recounting. This effect can be disconcerting to victims, and in children, may lead them to try to fill in the "gaps" with confabulations. This effect may be more marked if the child interprets an adult who is questioning them as disapproving of the "gaps" or disconnects. Children want to please adults, so they "fill in the gaps" accordingly. When this happens, the old danger of "detailing" comes into play, sidetracking real healing.

6. Traumatic memory, by nature, is often transferable. Especially in children, I have often noted that the well-known phenomenon of transference applies to abusive memories. There are many fine foster parents who have experienced the transferred accusations of abuse from foster children with PTSD. Believe it or not, this occasional transferring process is part of the child's healing. Trying to interpret and make sense of what has happened to them, the child may transfer not only emotion and psychic energy from the abuser to the foster parent, but direct accusation as well. This may be due to the fact that the foster parent has been understood by the child to be a safe (and strong) person to work through the emotions surrounding

the genuine abuse. There is a tendency in the field for such accusations to be reacted to by treatment teams quite dramatically, with investigations and moves from one foster home to another. While accusations of course need to be investigated with due diligence for the child's safety, they should also be understood as very real possibilities that are part and parcel to the care of such children, and a situation that could be used by the wise clinician as a springboard to progress for the child.

7. Traumatic memory, by nature, is often *evolving*. Traumatic memory is constantly evolving into a more manageable piece of baggage, one that is more *understood* by the victim, one that is less unwieldy to keep stored, and one that is lighter to bear. Time is needed for this evolution, and the pacing needs to be in the hands of the victim. Attributions as to causation, culpability, and the meanings of the events as well as interpretations of the outcomes for the victim are all evolutionary processes. The job of the clinician is to help the victim to navigate through the process and to avoid attributions that will negatively impact their life. This does not mean that such corrections to attributions need to be always made in the context of detailed memory; such corrections of attributions that have been internalized by the child (like self worth, being sullied, being lovable) should be addressed on a daily basis when they appear.

8. All memory is dependent upon the individual's developmental level, and must be approached with respect to that development. Each stage of development, as well as each individual, has unique aspects in the kinds of details that get encoded. For example, in an art museum visit, I may be emotionally overwhelmed by the collection of Impressionist paintings, while my ten year old son only recalls the picture of the man with a bandage on his ear. This means *all* development, intellectual, chronological maturity, moral and ethical development, and psychosexual development to name just a few. With young children, and especially young children who have experienced interpersonal trauma, there are more omissions of details than commission of false details (unless the child is being led by an adult to embellish with false details).

Many clinicians reading this text will have gotten their case once the child has been diagnosed with PTSD and the source of the PTSD (abuse) has been verified and already found appropriate disposition in the form of foster care or at least removal of the perpetrator from contact with the child. On the other hand, there may be those situations where abuse is revealed for the first time to the clinician in session with the child, or further abuse is reported concerning other perpetrators. There are many clinicians who do not work with children just because of such a conundrum. All clinicians of course, are mandated reporters, that is a given. But the usual question becomes; "how will my need to report the allegations impact the therapeutic alliance I have with the child…and how do I handle that fact?" That's a good question.

Experience tells me that when a child reveals to an adult, it is always intentional. The reveal may appear to be a "slip" or a "strong hint", but the reveal occurred for a reason. The very nature of telling someone who could help implies that there will be some kind of intervention. Children are bright enough to understand that their reveal will result in action; they are usually acutely aware of "child protective services".

It is my practice to immediately tell the child (in a gentle, age appropriate manner) that I in turn, will need to tell other people about what the child is saying. With younger children, I gently and respectfully state: "I'm sorry you were hurt. I don't think that children shout ever be hurt that way. I'm going to try hard to make it that you will never be hurt that way again by that person."

With older children, I begin the same, but directly state that I will need to report through the mandated channels, and what this entails. Even though the child has some rudimentary understanding of what their reveal will mean, they may begin to panic a bit following the reveal, and may need reassurance that their reveal is a positive step in their safety and happiness.

Generally speaking, if a child reveals information in a session that could have new legal implications, I do try to gain as much information (in a clearly Gentling fashion) as possible without leading, pressing, or pushing. My basic way of encouraging the child to continue to give me details is simple reflection of emotion, basic attending with eye contact, and small verbal encouragements ("mm-hmm, I see.") If the information given is enough of an indication of possible abuse, that is all I need to report to the mandated channels. I do not press a child to continue to give (possible) forensic details beyond their motivation to do so. This is neither my job nor, as I've already said, is it usually effective.

Though such a reveal and subsequent reporting response by the clinician surely impacts the intensity, original direction and progress of treatment, the fact that the child revealed to the clinician is a statement of therapeutic intimacy and trust. In most cases, this only serves to enhance treatment.

16 Understanding Secrets and Abuse

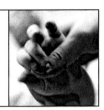

Perhaps the most apparent and culturally well known symptom of child abuse is that the child maintains the "secret" of the abuse for extended periods of time prior to revealing to any adult. This classic symptom does not disappear once a child initially reveals on his or her own, or their abuse is discovered due to obvious abuse physical injury. In many cases, the child has lived a majority, if not all of their life keeping multiple, difficult secrets concerning their abuse and family dysfunction.

Secrecy is just the first symptom noted by Dr. Roland Summit, who developed a descriptor of sexual abuse symptoms in children that he called the "Child Sexual Abuse Accommodation Syndrome." The reader who has experience with children who have been abused will recognize that the descriptors could also very well apply to abuses other than sexual:

- Secrecy about the abuse, reluctance to speak about it due to possible threats by the perpetrator.
- Emotional helplessness to resist or complain about the original abuse, or subsequent re-victimization by other perpetrators.
- Entrapment and accommodation, in that the child feels that there is no way to escape the abuse, so they learn to cope with it and adapt. The child's resolve to tell also may "fold" in the presence of the perpetrator or other persons associated with the perpetrator.
- Delayed, conflicted, and unconvincing disclosure of the abuse. This disclosure may seem exaggerated, inconsistent in detail, or simply vague.
- The child may "backpedal" or recant their allegations to restore the family structure, or to emotionally calm a parent, family member, or the perpetrator.

It is quite rare that a child who has been diagnosed with PTSD and who has been removed from the biological home has revealed *all* of the history of abuse that they have experienced to the child protection investigator. They likely have revealed just enough to buy them some temporary relief from abuse. What the child does not understand, of course, is that the resultant court decisions, based on the limited reveal and recommendations of the child protection agency, may be a very quick or eventual "return home goal". If the court and child protection agency does not have the full abuse history on record, the child may return home in very short order. As this threat of return becomes evident to the child, the child may decide to reveal yet another chunk of history, hoping that it will be enough to keep them out of the perpetration zone.

There is also the possible reality of an unspoken and/or unconscious contract between the child and the biological family/perpetrator that while *some* abuse detail has been given ("spilled the beans"), *particular details* are still contingent to follow-through of perpetrator threats. These threats classically are to either harm the children if they reveal, harm another loved one or pet, or to insure that if the child reveals, they will never have contact with a non-perpetrating family member. Thus, it becomes clear that the child's secrets carry with them some pretty heavy-duty baggage, and they must be addressed with care and gentleness, but also directly and realistically.

It would seem reasonable to also assert that for very young children, under the age of five, for example, who have been abused for all of their young lives, they are not so much as keeping a secret as simply failing to tell what is a common and mundane experience for them. As horrible as that sounds, a small child may not have enough life experience to have noticed or analyzed the fact that not all families work like theirs does.

Children will at times clearly state that they have a secret that they cannot tell, and may even state who told them to keep the secret. When this occurs, it can be a moment that raises a clinician's anxiety, and alters their countenance. I have witnessed fellow helpers become quite noticeably tense, begin to press the child for details, and have their vocal qualities become pressured.

Each of these characteristics may have a variety of sources, including anger at a perpetrator, fear for the child, or the natural excitement of hitting upon a clear and important issue in the child's treatment. The problem, of course, is that the child can *feel this shift* in the helper's countenance, and it may set off alarm bells for the child, which in turn shuts the child down. While there is the possibility that the child has made the "I have a secret" statement as way to begin to reveal, a helper's reactivity can make the child change their mind.

Another possibility of why the child has made the statement is in hopes that just revealing that they do have a secret will be enough to protect them. While a child may indeed have a secret, they may discover that their secret statement gets them a rapt attention from the helper, and may continue to use the statement in order to achieve and maintain that intense attention from an adult. Lastly, in family dynamics that genuinely have many secrets; the child may be so used to such a lifestyle that even insignificant things might be presented as a secret. Just because the child states that they have a secret, it may not be concerning abuse. The secret could range from Daddy's Meth lab in the garage to the birthday gift they plan to take to their cousin's party.

Once again, the clinician's gentle countenance becomes an important tool in dealing with "secret statements". There is a need for mindfulness about voice tone, body language, and the content of responses to the child's statement. Keeping an even, calm approach in such situations is not easy, of course, and even those of us that have been through this many times still experience near overwhelming emotions when the situation presents. The trick is to have been giving the child your best professional attending all the way to this point, and give the secret statement the same high level of attending that you have been presenting all along in treatment thus far. This will help to alleviate any obvious shift in your attention, intensity, and emotion.

This is not to say, of course, that you express *no* emotion. Expressing curiosity about the "secret" is entirely appropriate, as is demonstrating concern that the secret may be something troubling the child. In the area of content, it is a good idea to convey two important ideas to the child in such a situation.

First, that you know about two kinds of secrets: good secrets (like surprise birthday parties) and bad secrets (like someone hurting a child). Secondly, there is a need to convey to the child that if they have a bad secret, you cannot help them if they do not tell what the secret is. Below are three vignettes to illustrate the points about secrets thus far made:

Tae, Age five

Tae, age five, is on the floor of the foster home, playing with action figures. The clinician joins him. Tae begins to bang two action figures together in an aggressive fashion, and shouts: "You bitch! Get offa me right now, or I'm gonna pop you!" Startled by such language from a young child, the clinician states: "Wow, they are angry at each other, what are they angry at?" Tae responds: "They are mad at each other and want to fight." The clinician asks if Tae has ever seen two people that angry and want to fight before. Tae nods his head 'yes', then states: "I have a secret." The clinician's ears perk up, and he begins to attend to Tae closer, shifting to more consistent eye contact, and leaning forward a bit. "What is your secret?" the clinician asks. "I can't tell." says Tae. The clinician, not allowing any time between Tae's statement and the clinicians' response states: "You need to tell if someone has hurt you. Who hurt you? What did they do?" Tae visibly changes from a relatively open posture to one that is much more closed: he pulls his action figures into his lap, looks down at the floor, and his facial expression becomes flat. The clinician senses that he is on to something important, and states: "If something bad has happened to you, you need to tell me right now." Tae looks up, but does not give eye contact. He states: "Nobody hurt me, can I go get a snack now?"

Laura, Age Seven

In session with Laura, age seven, the clinician has been trying to help Laura begin to work through emotions surrounding her removal from her home due to alleged neglect issues. Laura's mother had been arrested for drug possession and there are suspicions that the mother was prostituting for money. While playing with dolls, Laura begins to simulate sex acts between the dolls. The clinician asks, in a calm and curious manner, what the dolls are doing. Laura just shrugs, and then asks the clinician if she can tell the clinician a secret. The clinician responds quickly, with a constricted voice telling Laura that she can tell the clinician "anything...*anything.*" Laura leans to the clinician, cupping her hand to the clinician's ear in a classic secret motion, and whispers: "I got my sister a doll just like this one for her birthday, next week." Feeling slightly let down, the clinician's posture slumps, and states flatly: "Oh, that's a nice gift."

David, Age Seven

David, age seven, was removed from the care of his mother, along with a younger sibling, because of neglect. There is suspicion by the treatment team that David had also been sexually abused by the mother's paramour, who is now out of the home and broken up with David's mother. David has consistently demonstrated sexualized behaviors in the foster home.

David recently had pulled down his pants in front of another child in the foster home and allegedly said to the other child "suck it." The clinician is hoping to address the behavior with David, who had been sent to his room last evening by his foster parents following the incident. After greetings, the clinician tells David in a gentle, but firm and direct way that the foster parents have told him what happened last night.

David, usually having a bright affect, flattens and hangs his head. The clinician, again with a very gentle and firm voice, states to David that he is not in trouble with the clinician, but wants to help David. The clinician, citing fairness and accuracy, invites David to tell what happened in his own words. David says, still with his head down: "Yea, I did it. I told Jeremy to suck me."

The clinician pauses, allowing the statement to settle, and giving time for David to continue. David remains silent, but glances up at the clinician. "I wonder why you said that and pulled your pants down," stated the clinician in a low, even tone.

There is another long pause. David says quietly, as he begins to cry: "I have a secret I can't tell."

"Mmm…that kind of secret is difficult" states the clinician, and pauses again. David repeats that he cannot tell. The clinician responds: "Well, you don't *have* to tell me, but it sounds like you might feel better if you did." David states, almost as if he has memorized the line: "If I tell, she gets hurt."

Easily reading between the lines, but not pushing the process, the clinician simply reflects both emotion and content: "Telling this bad secret might mean that someone you care about gets hurt, and that scares you." There is another long pause, and the clinician gets a box of tissues and hands them to David, who takes one and blows his nose.

The clinician states quietly to David that he wants to help David, but the secret may be standing in the way of that. The silence continues. David picks up a crayon and begins to color in a coloring book, and says: "Maybe later." The clinician picks up a crayon and begins to color the opposite page. David begins to chat about his upcoming school year.

It is clear to the clinician that David is finished talking about the secret for now. But that is OK, the clinician understands the wisdom of being patient, firm, and gentle in such situations. Today's movement in treatment is very significant, because it is the first time David has even hinted at the fact that he had been sexually abused by his mother's paramour.

It must be remembered that while children are very resilient, they experience even small increments of therapeutic intensity surrounding the secret of abuse as very intense; much more so than we helpers might calculate. While in other forms of therapy, the clinician may use an increasing intensity technique to illustrate a point or press for movement in treatment; this is generally counterproductive in abuse cases.

17   When a Person is a Known Trigger

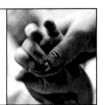

Social interaction and response is, of course, activated by exposure of one person to another. In this sense, everyone is 'triggered' by others that they have contact with daily. A chance meeting of a friend in the community, or an irritating phone solicitation can create specific memories and emotions. So too, in a magnified manner, for victims who come into contact with a person that triggers their memory of one of their critical incidents.

When a person is a trigger to a child's stress reactions, it is usually quite clear from anecdotal evidence. The person who serves as a trigger may not necessarily be a perpetrator of abuse against the child, but is quite often someone who is fairly close to the child, such as a family member. In addition, of course, any actual perpetrator may be a strong and reliable trigger to stress reactivity in a child. The situation can become quite complex, with the child's stress reactivity having different intensity expression in relation to different people who are triggers to the stress behaviors.

When a person (or multiple persons) is suspected as being a trigger for a child, stressed behavior needs to begin to be tracked and evaluated in correlation to the child's contact with the suspected person-triggers. More detail concerning what data to gather, how to analyze, arrange, and present it is the subject of the next chapter. This information, primarily of concern for direct treatment, may become quite important as evidence to child protective services and courts as to why contact between the child and the triggering person should be controlled and managed in order to allow treatment to progress.

In situations where, for example, a child has been abused by one parent, but not abused by the other, the child will likely have a clear and reliable presentation of a stress behavior set in relation to the offending parent, and may have a milder reaction to the other parent, who presumably should have been protecting the child from the abuser. The same effect may extend to sibling contact with the identified

PTSD diagnosed child: if the abused child is the older of the siblings, and willingly placed themselves (or sacrificed themselves, as it were) between the younger child and the perpetrator to protect the younger child, the abused child may have stress reactivity upon exposure to the sibling they protected.

These dynamics obviously become more complex when there are more people involved that make up the family structure that the abused child has been living in. These multiple dyads, triads, and alliances all need to be considered if the child (and clinician) is having regular contact with the family of the victim. In most cases, if interpersonal abuse has occurred in the family, the family as a whole likely needs treatment for their ongoing dysfunctions. Though the focus of this book is towards individual treatment of an abused, traumatized child living away from the offending family, a clinician may find himself or herself treating the child who continues to live in the household that was the abuse context. In such cases, the wise clinician may want to insist on a team effort in the family.

It is important to re-state that just because a child has a stress reaction to contact with a person, it does not necessarily follow that that person is a perpetrator. This is a special temptation when the person triggering the child is an adult. A child may be highly reactive to an adult who was either present or nearby when the abuse occurred, and did little or nothing to stop the assault. Or, the adult was unresponsive or admonishing when the child approached them for help following the assault. Though a trigger person may not be a perpetrator, when a trigger person is identified, it should bring up a 'red flag' to the clinician, and the clinician should explore the reasons why the person is a trigger to the child.

18 The Family Preservation Bias

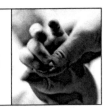

Educating Caregivers: Foster Parents, Teachers, CYS, and Judges

A serious challenge to work progress with abused, stress disordered children, is that the courts and child protective agencies often maintain very strong "family preservation" biases that continue to force the child to be exposed to a family member who is either a strong trigger, or is the actual perpetrator. This complaint is not to suggest that once abuse has been founded, that child should never have contact with the perpetrating family member, but it does mean that the intensity and depth of the child's stressed behavior set should be the guiding factor in contact, not a misplaced effort to maintain the parent-child bond. If child's bond with their perpetrating parent has been so damaged that the child has a PTSD diagnosis as a result, the child's individual healing needs to take priority. Trying to maintain the bond under such conditions is like trying to put a band-aid over a gapping chest wound.

Treatment can certainly reunify a family, even including a perpetrator, but this clinician is of the opinion that repeated, intense and deep reactions to contact between the child and triggering family members not only inhibits the child's ability to heal, but may also inhibit the perpetrator's motivation to progress in their own remedial and healing process. The task is to control and manage any contact between the traumatized child and the triggering people (especially a known perpetrator) in their life.

A rather common effect that is often missed by those professionals who only have occasional contact with the child and family (such as child protective staff, as opposed to clinicians who may have weekly or more than weekly contact) is that when the child is observed during visitation with triggering family members, the child may *appear* to be quite cheerful, positive, unafraid, and affectionate. Once again, the extended treatment team needs to recall the lessons of Child Sexual Abuse Accommodation Syndrome: the child's behaviors may, in fact, adapt and accommodate the context of the visit, and who is present at the visit. In most cases, the child protective caseworker is not present for the twenty four to seventy two hours following the visit, wherein the child's stress reactivity behavior set is likely to present in a fairly strong fashion.

Even a casual probing of a foster parent will reveal that foster children have clearly different behavioral expressions following contact or visit with biological family members. This is not to say that the highly stressed behavior sets always occur to the same intensity, frequency, or duration following contact, but they do occur. Over the course of treatment of the child, if treatment is moving according to plan, reactivity behavior sets should be measurably lessened, even to the point of being extinguished.

In severe cases, where stress reactivity is very intense, and takes a long time to settle, there may be a need to request a halt to all contact with the triggering biological family member from child protective services and the court. 'Severe' means that the child's high level of allostatic load and expression disallows the child to have any recovery time between contacts. In effect, the child does not return to any homeostasis either physiologically or emotionally between visits.

Typically, child protective service agencies and courts have a minimum required level of visitation, in many cases weekly or every other week. There have been many cases in my experience that the child has just barely regained a sense of calm and routine before being told of yet another visit. Effective healing and treatment of the child cannot take place in a context of the intense, repeated stress reactions this implies. This said, stopping contact between a child and biological family members is a prescription that should only be done with the greatest consideration, compassion, and adequate behavioral study proofs that is genuinely in the child's best interest.

Cessation of contact between the child and the triggering family member is not permanent; it is a temporary measure to allow the child to have time to heal and build ego strength, as well as gain some stress inoculation skills. My experiences tell me that a moratorium on contact needs to be tailored to the levels of reactivity in the child; some children may need total contact removal (visits, phone calls, mailings), while other children may be able to tolerate phone contacts. The clinician needs to have the ability to adjust contacts to a level that the child is able to tolerate without experiencing moderate to severe stress reactions. The tactic then is to slowly increase the kinds, duration, and frequency of contacts at a level that the child can continue to tolerate.

If the extended treatment team decides to curtail contact, the family member(s) who are triggers need to be told about this in a compassionate and sensitive manner. This is a painful turn of events for any family member, to be told that someone is altering or taking away your ability to see your child, grandchild, or sibling. Informing of the decision may fall to someone specific on the team other than the clinician, but if it is the clinician that has made the prescription, then it should be the same clinician who informs the parent.

It is helpful if the clinician has experience in grief and mourning therapy, because this is essentially what will occur for the triggering family member. If the clinician does not have experience in this area, they are not off the hook; they should educate themselves in therapeutic skills in helping people with loss and grief. Unlike death, of course, the cessation of contact is only temporary, and the triggering family member(s) should be apprised of the plan that has been made of how long the moratorium on contact will be, and what the reunification strategy will be.

As someone who has made these kinds of prescriptions and informed parents many times, I can attest to how difficult and uncomfortable the process is. The clinician needs to be prepared for a full range of reaction from the triggering person, including not only tears but anger and rage as well. It is my practice to be sure to have on hand a written page detailing the reasons why the visits are being so radically changed, so that I can give the person a chance, when they become calmer, to later read about what I have just told them. It is a very good idea to be clear about inviting the person to call you about any questions they have about the temporary halt in contact, or to enquire about the progress of the child.

Anecdotal evidence suggests that some stress disordered children, under some conditions, may transfer their stress reactivity behaviors (in the sense of a person being a trigger) from the original person or cluster of people to someone who is secondary in their lives. This may be some other caregiver, teacher, coach, or even a clinical interventionist. The case vignette below illustrates this point:

> Danny is seven years old and struggling with his stress reactivity at school. He is the victim of both physical and sexual abuse by a legal guardian who was a close friend of Danny's father and agreed to take Danny in until the father could clear up some legal and substance abuse issues. While in the guardian's care, Danny was abused and neglected, including one critical incident where the guardian placed a handgun to Danny's head, and subsequently wrestled him into a closet and then locked it. Danny is now in foster care, and has been doing well in integrating into the foster home. He clearly feels safe there, and demonstrates this by having few stress episodes in the home.

However, Danny is a royal terror in school; he acts out by ripping posters off of walls, screaming obscenities, hitting and pushing other children, and pulling out his own hair. Danny's Therapeutic Support Staff (TSS) is at his wit's end. Nothing the

TSS does seems to help. The clinician who guides the TSS had put restraint measures in place about two months ago, and there is an average of three restraints lasting five minutes each per day. It seems as if Danny just keeps getting more extreme in his reactivity. But curiously, the TSS reports that when he was off for two days due to illness and a substitute TSS took over, Danny had two relatively good days. But within one minute of the TSS return into the school room, Danny became aggressive and vulgar.

Danny's reactivity and behaviors towards the presence of this TSS are quite understandable. The clinician has made a basic error in treatment of a child with PTSD as a result of interpersonal violence. The usefulness of this TSS has long been over; the first restraint likely ensured that. If the child is bright, he might associate the TSS with the clinician, equally ending the clinician's effectiveness as well.

19   Stress Behavior Data Collection

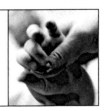

The reader will recall the Child Stress Profile (CSP), and its use as a means to discover a child's unique stress behavior pattern, and as a tool to measure progress and outcomes of treatment. In addition to these uses, the Stress Profile can be used to extrapolate the major behavioral signs and symptoms (those in the 'intense" range) as a means to begin to discern if and how *particular people*, as well as environmental cues in the child's life are serving as triggers to the behaviors.

By making a simple list of the items on the CSP that are in the "intense" range, the clinician can form a reference for the caregiver/foster parent to use to track daily stress episodes. A simple form may look like the one below:

Child's Name:_____   **Date:** _____

Time of day/duration: **Intensity:** mild moderate severe (circle one)

Possible or Known Trigger:

Behavioral Signs:

In order to help the caregiver to gauge intensity of the behavioral sign, the clinician should assist the caregiver in describing the most intense stress episode that has been yet observed, along with a stress episode that just barely gets the caregiver's attention that something is amiss with the child. This then becomes the relative measure of intensity.

As the reader can see, from this simple data form can be gleaned much useful information, including developing a larger view of any rhythms of stress episodes, possible anniversary reactions, identification of any new trigger information, and possibly revelation of unique and subtle behavioral 'tells' that could be useful in heading off an episode. It should be noted that the data form is also a useful tool in gathering dynamic information about the caregiver: their consistency and detailing in entering data and their relative level of stress in relation to the child.

For example, it is a good habit to review the data with the caregiver on a regular basis. If there is a consistent rating and high number of daily "moderate to severe" episodes, it may be an indication of not only the child's stress, but the caregiver's as well. Follow up interventions for the caregiver, if this is the case, will be well within the clinician's skills.

A second extrapolation from the Stress Profile Tool is use the list of "intense" behavioral signs as a checklist for the caregiver to fill out following contacts between the child and biological family members (or others associated with the family). The caregiver can be instructed to place a "24", "48" or "72" before or after the behavioral signs that the child demonstrates prior to or after a contact with people suspected to be triggers. The idea is to indicate if a symptom presents and persists within 24-72 hours before or following contact.

An abbreviated example of such a simple data form appears below:

Time Before Behavior	Behavior	Time After Behavior
24	Hiding food	24, 48
	Flat affect	24, 48
24	Hypervigilant	24, 48, 72
	⋮	
	.	

This data then becomes useful in informing the treatment team how to manage and control contacts. An acceptable level of reactivity is established; perhaps one that lasts only 24 hours in 90% of the behaviors prior to and following a contact. Once that level is achieved consistently, then the frequency, duration, and intensity (as in number of triggering people in the contact, context of contact, etc.) can be increased, with the same expectation of low reactivity. Should the child's stress reactivity rise in response to an increase in contact, visitation then can be backed off accordingly.

The data can also be used to identify whom the child is reactive to. Visitations can be separated to include only one suspected triggering person at a time, in order to ascertain which person the child is most reactive to. Again the reader is admonished not to necessarily conclude that this person with the highest reactivity rating is a perpetrator of abuse, even though this is often the case.

It is very useful for treatment purposes and for presentation to child protective services when making a prescription to curtail contact to translate the data into graph form in order to illustrate the correlation between the child's contact with a person and the child's intensified stress reaction behaviors. The child protective agency tires to make a case to the courts as to the advisability of the child's return to the people and home where the abuse took place; this kind of data helps them to make that case. A sample Stress Behavior Summary Sheet appears on the next page. Please see Appendix D for blank copies of all the forms in this chapter.

Janie Doe

Stress Behavior Summary Sheet

JAN. '07 — stress behaviors rated Severe, Moderate, Mild. (Days 1–31)

Date	Severe	Moderate	Mild	Contact	Number of incidents	duration
1	▓			V	X 1	7 h
2		▓				
3				C		
4		▓	▓		4	3 h
5		▓	▓		4	4 h
6						
7						
8						
9		▓	▓		1	1 h
10		▓	▓	C	2	1 h
11		▓	▓		1	1 h
12						
13						
14	▓	▓	▓		2	8 h
15	▓	▓	▓	V	2	9 h
16	▓	▓	▓		X 2	1 h
17	▓	▓	▓	C	1	1 h
18	▓	▓	▓	C		
19	▓	▓	▓	V	X	8 h
20	▓	▓	▓		X	1 h
21		▓	▓		2	2 h
22						
23						
24				C		
25						
26	▓			V	X	6 h
27			▓		1	1 h
28						
29						
30						
31				C		

Mild, Moderate, Severe are rated according to the intensity, quality, and duration of specific stress signs presented.

V=visit   P=phone contact   M=missed or cancelled contact
X= multiple   T=Clinician visit   C=Child Protection caseworker visit

Notes: 19th and 20th: family taking down holiday decorations, Janie thought family was moving

While the data collection and analysis process as presented here is quite straight-forward, it is a bit more complicated than first glance. In most cases, visits between the child and biological members include multiple family members and possibly multiple visit locations. The clinician may need to gain the support of the child protective agency and the court to arrange for separate visits between the child and individual family members in order to ascertain if there is *one particular family member* that is the trigger for the stress reactivity in the child. Caution must be used to schedule these visitations at least one week apart, so that one visit reaction does not contaminate the other.

Such extensive efforts are worth pursuit: I have had many cases that this strategy has identified one particular person in the child's family that served to be the most intense and significant trigger. In addition, I have also discovered that it can help clear a person as a trigger for the child, as is illustrated in the vignette below:

Shelly, Age Seven

Shelly is a seven year old girl who had lived with her maternal grandmother for the past two years because her father had been jailed for drugs, and her mother was generally neglectful of Shelly and her older sister, age ten, and her older brother, age nine. Shelly's mother and the mother's new paramour had taken care of the children for some six months in the past year, but the children were returned to the grandmother because the child protective agency had gotten involved with the mother and paramour due to reports from the children's school about neglect and the children's oppositional behaviors.

Subsequently, while the mother of the children and her paramour were visiting the grandmother and children, the grandmother discovered that the paramour was sexually abusing Shelly. Since Shelly's behaviors deteriorated following this discovery, she was placed by the protection agency in foster care.

There, she began to reveal a long pattern of sexual abuse by the paramour and her biological father that not only involved her, but her sister and brother as well. Later, there was evidence that the paramour and the children's mother participated in placing nude images of the children on the internet for profit. The courts soon ended contact between the children and their mother, and the paramour was charged and jailed.

Following several months of treatment in the foster home, it was discovered that the weekly visits between Shelly and her grandparents and siblings was triggering moderate to severe reactions upon return to the foster home that lasted from twenty four to seventy two hours. The clinician decided to arrange for visits to be made with only the grandmother at first, and then the siblings and other family members were added.

In addition, visits were taken out of the grandmother's home and done in the community. The data collected clearly illustrated that while Shelly was mildly to moderately reactive to family members such as her grandmother and siblings, her reaction were far greater when the visits took place in the grandmother's home; presumably because some of the sexual abuse took place there.

This data allowed the treatment team to focus treatment for Shelly; more community visits, less in home visits, and when in-home visits occur, the counselor can be explicit about the home, the cues, and the triggers with Shelly. A slow and measured de-sensitization and work at establishing the grandmother's home as a now safe place could begin.

The importance of behavioral data in these kinds of cases cannot be underestimated; it can focus treatment, demonstrate cue and trigger connections, give evidence needed to curtail contacts between the victim and people who are strong and reliable triggers, and give direction to the overall healing process.

20 Classroom Protocols

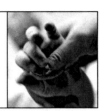

School presents a special set of challenges for the clinician. Schools and individual teachers vary in their understandings and attitudes towards mental health issues and services, as well as the sources and approaches to children's behaviors. The variables include the experience level of the teacher, the teacher and school administration's experience of mental health professionals before your arrival in their school, and all of the prevailing trends and attitudes towards special needs children that sometimes have a regional flavor.

As stated earlier, some people have a very difficult time in letting go of preconceived notions and adopting new gestalts about the source and nature of a child's 'misbehaviors'. Teacher and school administrators are no different. The clinician will find some educators very open to learning (no pun intended) about Acute Stress and Post Traumatic Stress and the most effective ways to help a child gain new positive behaviors. But other educators may have a very difficult time accepting that the behavior that they are experiencing from the child is not simple oppositional behavior that needs the correct amount of pressure to change. Still others may exacerbate the child's plight by calling in the parent-perpetrator to take the parent to task as to why their child is not well disciplined. This, of course, is a disaster for the child.

Although the highly open educator or school is rare, the educator and school that totally rejects the premises presented in this book is equally rare. In most cases, the teacher and school lie somewhere between the two extremes. The clinician's first task is to understand how the *school protocol* works in relation to mental health services. Each district (and in turn, school in the district) may have a different protocol for how a clinician is to gain access to the school, classroom, and child when direct intervention or treatment is needed. A good rule of thumb is to avoid wasting time going to the school on an initial visit, and make a phone call to the correct staff member. Most schools have a phone voicemail system, and the child's teacher is good place to start. This call should be focused on asking the teacher about the school and district protocol for having needed access to the classroom to observe the child, and access to one on one work with the child in the school environment. Whatever the protocol is, follow it.

The second task is to probe the pertinent school staff and ascertain their openness to gaining more understanding of the child, the child's diagnosis, and the Gentling approach. It is taken for granted that the clinician has gained all of the needed releases to discuss such issues with school staff. It is best not to push too hard in this probing phase, as this can make the job of educating the school staff more difficult later on. This is a time to be conscious of making use of your clinical joining skills, especially with the classroom teacher.

A varied approach to providing education to the school staff is desirable. All of the clinician's references to the child should make use of the language specific to the Gentling Approach. How we speak about the stress disordered child, and using the proper terms related to the disorder is a teaching effort towards everyone we meet in connection with the case. A second form of education can be to provide well written literature about Acute Stress and PTSD as it related to child victims of interpersonal abuse. In my work, I offer the school staff my card, pointing out my professional website, that has an 'articles' page where they can read about stress disorders in children and the Gentling Approach at their convenience.

Assuming that the proper releases have been gained, the clinician should also apprise the classroom teacher (as well as other needed school administrators) of the course of likely presence of the clinician in the classroom. This is professional courtesy. In addition, the teacher should also be apprised of the purpose and results of the clinician's in class behavioral observations of the child. While it is never advisable to interrupt a class to chat with the teacher, there should be an appropriate time arranged where the clinician can have a few words with the teacher either in person or by phone, for intermittent updates of the in school efforts that the clinician is involved with.

Key in the effort to help the child to lower in school symptoms and behaviors related to their stress disorder is the clinician's involvement in the development and reviews of the Individualized Education Plan, if the child has one. If the child does not have an IEP, and the clinician is seeing clear stress behavior problems that are interfering with the child's education, then an evaluation for Emotional Support should be recommended. In the behavioral plan portions of the IEP, the clinician can be very helpful in steering the developed interventions in a fashion that is as close as possible to the Gentling Approach.

Being prepared to hand busy, pertinent school staff a one-sheet 'suggestion list' can be a productive way of engaging the school staff in wanting to learn more about how they can help the child. This should always be followed up on at a later date to see if the staff has questions about the material on the list. Should the clinician finds a person who is highly interested in learning more about stress disorders in children who have suffered interpersonal trauma, take a few extra moments and *teach* them. And by all means, refer them to this book! A sample 'quick teach sheet' appears on the following two pages.

[QT1] Suggestions to School Staff for a Stress Disordered Student)

1. Learn about stress disorders in children. Acute Stress Disorder and Post Traumatic Stress Disorder are the most common severe forms of stress in children, but children without these diagnosed disorders may also exhibit stress signs.

2. Learn the individual child's signs of stress. Each child exhibits stress differently. Many children get labeled as "oppositional" or "attention deficit", but are really expressing stress signs. Some children become forgetful, needy, clingy, and generally regressed in their behaviors. Stress disorders often mimic other disorders; the key is that approaches used for the other disorders do not work with stress disordered children.

3. Watch for and help the child avoid or be extracted quickly from stressful situations, such as peer conflict or intense over stimulation. Do not press a child for answers to academic questions if they clearly are having trouble recalling the information.

4. Provide opportunities for "stress breaks". These can be for the whole class such as brief stretch and exercise sessions, quiet time, meditation, listening to recorded nature sounds, etc. Or, you can send the stressed child out to carry a "message" to another teacher or the office (opportunity for quiet in the hallway is key). It is ideal for a stress disordered child to have a very quiet place to be able to retreat to when you notice their stress level is moderately high (don't wait until it is high, because they *will* begin to act out).

5. To avoid abuse of any needed "stress breaks", set a clear limit on the number and time allowed.

6. If the child becomes emotionally needy or clingy: arrange for another staff member in the building to provide brief, regular "nurture" breaks for the child. These can be simply checking on the child's day, helping them clarify or talk about their mood, perhaps sharing a sticker or other treat for having a good (morning, afternoon, day), or a few moments to cuddle a stuffed animal or attend to the classroom animal.

7. Children with stress disorders may have memory and concentration problems. They likely know the material, but when stressed, cannot recall. Offer more time. Do not press and demand, just encourage. Offer to take a stress break and come back to the task later. Remember that what may not seem demanding to you may be terribly demanding to the child. Create a method of sending home a homework memo to the parents regularly, or have a

"communication notebook". Provide an extra quiet and private space for work to be done.

8. A child with stress disorder will often "rush" through assignments and tasks. This is a sign that they are stressed. High stress "dims" the child's ability to learn and do tasks proficiently. Their "rushing" is a form of "flight", which is common in stressed children. They are not being lazy, or have attention deficit problems, they are stressed. Help the child by either accepting or interrupting the work and providing a stress break. Let them return to the work when they are less stressed.

9. Stress disordered children may be disorganized. They may need extra help and time in keeping their school materials in order, or recognizing schedules. A simple daily/weekly schedule on their desk or locker can help this.

10. Stress disordered children need more affirmation, guidance, and praise than other children. They often are insecure and cannot self evaluate very well, so adults need to offer more frequent assessments (especially positive ones.)

21 Self-Care for the Clinician or the Differentiated Helper

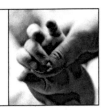

Treating and caring for victims of Acute and Post Traumatic Stress is a wearing, tiring, and sometimes painful endeavor. Hearing children's stories of their critical incidents, and even being aware of the incidents through the child's history can impact the clinician's daily experience in some weighty ways. There is plenty of research that has shown how 'compassion fatigue' operates, and the corresponding symptoms. Beyond compassion fatigue, a clinician who works consistently and closely with child victims of personal trauma can begin to experience symptoms of Acute and Post Traumatic Stress to a considerable degree.

This contagion effect of stress symptoms is also well researched; it is well known, for example, that a child who witnesses their mother being abused (and who has not been physically touched by a perpetrator) can develop stress symptoms similar to ones that their mother develops (secondary traumatization). This truth needs to cause the clinician to do frequent self-checks for symptoms and signs within themselves, and then to take remedial measures. If the clinician works with foster parents who care for the child, they also need to become aware and coached concerning this effect and the methods of self care.

Each and every contact or work session with a stress disordered child should be de-briefed in the clinician's own mind. It's a good idea to review the content of the session of course, but even more importantly, review your own emotions. All too often, clinicians take for granted that they are able to 'turn off the clinical switch' when they complete a work session. This is not always so; sometimes we only *think* we switched it off. We may have in fact fallen into the basic trap of the disorder: just try to forget about it, and then it will go away.

Clinicians are taught to keep distance from the client for many reasons: to be more effective, to remain objective, to control transference and countertransference. The plain truth is that when the client is a small child, and the substance of the work to be done has to do with abuse, our ability to maintain this space is more difficult, and at times, impossible. Clinicians are, by nature, very empathetic people. Empathy too, has an important place in treatment, but it makes us vulnerable to 'catching' the child's pain.

Therefore, making this self-debriefing a routine process is a key idea. Allow yourself to *really feel* the pain, sadness, fear, anger, rage, and confusion of the child during your post session meditation. If you feel the need to yell, clench your fists, or cry, do so. Sometimes simply sitting with the sadness that is created can be an effective tool. A side-effect of working with stress disordered children is that the clinician may dream about the child, or the abuse situation that the child has experienced. This is a telling clue that the clinician may not be taking care of themselves well enough, or if it occurs infrequently, may just be a way of our unconscious to process the emotions we have concerning the case.

Having the support of others is very important in avoiding burn out. Colleagues can provide not only clinical consultation, but also emotional and cognitive process-sing consultation on trauma cases. Family and friends, while not privy to identities and details of the child or the content of the session work, are also important supports for the clinician. Family and friends should be educated in the signs of stress disorder transference as a safeguard for the clinician. We may not be able to always see ourselves clearly enough to know that we are showing signs of this kind of stress, and others around us can give us a nudge.

Beyond these, maintaining sensible and basic self care habits like eating right, getting enough sleep, exercise, and setting aside time to enjoy a full range of activities and relationships that have nothing to do with the work is a final defense against burnout. I personally find my involvement in my hobbies to be a most effective de-stressor.

22 Sample Treatment Plan

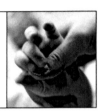

The brief goal plan below is a basic outline of one that I frequently use in my daily work. Quite frequently, children with other issues as well, and separate goal for managing anger and aggression or teaching assertiveness or peer social skills would be added to make a more complete treatment plan. The reader is welcome to copy and use the material here for their own cases.

Goal #1: Bill will become as comfortable as possible with his divided family situation and history of abuse.

Baseline: Bill has demonstrated signs of adjustment problems in being in foster care. He has also demonstrated behavioral signs of high stress reactivity as related to his history of abuse and abuse exposure.

Long Term Goal: Bill will be able to learn and consistently use the skills needed to end his observed signs and stated symptoms of discomfort and dysfunction, as evidenced by a reduction of 5 items from the current 62 items in the intense range on the Child Stress Profile.

1A Measurable Objective: Bill will learn and consistently use a positive engagement/processing method to help him relieve problematic signs and symptoms, as demonstrated by his positive engagement and processing in three out of four treatment sessions for one full month of (4) sessions.

Expected Outcome: Bill will learn how to engage in a cognitive-behavioral approach to treatment for his current issues.

Specific Interventions/persons responsible: Clinician will teach Bill how to recognize his own symptoms and behavioral signs as well as methods to block, interrupt, or mange the symptoms of stress outlined in the Child Stress Profile. Various approaches and methods will be used to attain the goal, including cognitive-behavioral, Gentling, therapy homework, and play interactions and desensitization in home, school, and community environments. Bill will receive verbal praise for his prompted and spontaneous use of the learned skills. Bill will not be pressed to relate details of his abuse episodes, but should he spontaneously decide to relate these, the team members will listen, empathize, and support him in processing.

1B Measurable Objective: Bill and his current caregivers (home(s), school staff, and Therapeutic Support Staff) will learn and consistently use designed interventions, based on behavioral observations, when Bill has a stress episode related to his divided family or history of abuse.

Expected Outcome: Consistent and effective external support by caregivers when Bill is in a stress episode.

Specific Interventions/persons responsible: Clinician will teach Bill and his caregivers on how to recognize stressed symptoms and behavioral signs as well as methods to block, interrupt, or mange the symptoms of stress outlined in the Child Stress Profile. Various approaches and methods will be used to attain the goal, including education, cognitive-behavioral, Gentling, therapy homework, and play interactions and desensitization in home, school, and community environments where he has access to interactions with peers. Bill's caregivers will keep a journal to document their use and observations of his signs and reported symptoms. Bill will cooperate with a weekly review of the symptoms and signs each week with the clinician.

Postscript

My experiences with abused children with PTSD have been a burden and a joy; I wouldn't trade them for anything. It is my sincere hope that the reader will also come to the conclusion that helping a child to reshape their life after interpersonal abuse is a deeply rewarding experience.

There is still so much for me (and you) to learn and do. I want to figure out how to heal a child's damaged sexuality following experiences of sexual abuse. I want to find the means to do an outcomes study on Gentling. I want to produce workbooks for children and adults on abuse and PTSD recovery. I want to hear from those of you who have used Gentling successfully (and not successfully). One thing is for certain: the children will continue to show me the way.

Appendix A: Child Stress Profile

W.E.Krill, Jr. M.S.P.C.

Child's Name:_____   Date:_____

Name of interviewer:_____

Interviewees:

Name:_____ Relationship_____

Name:_____ Relationship_____

Name:_____ Relationship_____

Directions: For each sign that the child demonstrates, rate that sign.

Scoring for each item: one of the 3 choices from the grid or "D" for *Does Not Appear*

Symptom is...	Not Frequent	Frequent
Not Intense		*FN*
Intense	*NI*	*FI*

Question: *Does the child....*	Score
1. Does the child have repeated hits from multiple stressors in their history?	
2. Does the child currently receive hits from intense stressors?	
3. Does the child struggle to adapt to novel situations?	
4. Does the child demonstrate a prolonged stress response?	
5. Does the child have an inadequate response to danger, threat, or injury?	
6. Does the child overreact to small events?	
7. Does the child underreact to large events?	
8. Does the child startle easily?	
9. Does the child demonstrate unexplained hyperarousal?	
10. Does the child have a difficult time calming down when upset or excited?	
11. Does the child become verbally aggressive with little provocation?	
12. Does the child run away or hide when they feel threatened?	
13. Does the child's pupils dilate, eyes get "glassy"?	
14. Does the child facial expressions become flat when upset?	
15. Does the child seem to "freeze" when threatened?	
16. Does the child demonstrate stress reactions prior to or after contact with people associated with the trauma?	
17. Does the child eat very fast, or over eat to the point of being sick?	
18. Does the child always seem to be watchful, vigilant, or overly cautious?	
19. Does the child appear "zombie-like" when upset?	
20. Does the child regress in behaviors when upset? (whine, cry, suck thumb, wet/soil self)	
21. Does the child have a hard time telling you what they are thinking or feeling when upset?	
22. Does the child seem to be upset (agitated) one moment, and fine (calm) the next?	
23. Does the child appear to have forgotten about the stress episode they just went through?	
24. Does the child fail to recall what upset him/her after a stress episode is over?	
25. Does the child seem to be upset for long periods of time?	
26. Does the child go to sleep following a stress episode?	
27. Does the child stay upset, agitated, and hyperactive for more than a whole day?	
28. Does the child verbalize about trauma memories at times that are out of context?	

29. Does the child show emotion when relating these memories?	
30. Does the child verbalize traumatic memories and expressed little or no emotion?	
31 Does the child. have any places, situations, or items that seem to trigger a stress reaction in the child (if yes, list).	
32. Does the child point out real scars or areas where no visible injury exists and complain about pain?	
33. Does the child have nightmares?	
34. Does the child ever speak to you about the nightmare? (if yes, please list content)	
35. Does the child simulate or act out sex acts?	
36. Does the child become emotional with you or someone else, and it seems as if it has to do with someone else? (transference)	
37. Does the child ever seem to be daydreaming and become emotional?	
38. Does the child seem to have very fragile emotions?	
39. Does the child re-enact known content from a trauma in play?	
40. Does the child ever speak to people who are not there? (hallucination)	
41. Does the child have any anniversary reactions? (if so, please list)	
42. Does the child flinch at simple touch?	
43. Does the child hide items, food, soiled clothing, or themselves?	
44. Does the child speak about or use names of known perpetrators when highly stressed?	
45. Does the child actively or passively avoid talking about their trauma or people associated with it?	
46. Does the child actively or passively avoid contact with people or places associated with the trauma?	
47. Does the child have times where they refuse affection or comfort attempts?	
48. Does the child lack empathy for others?	
49. Does the child bully or victimize others?	
50. Does the child harm animals?	
51. Does the child play with fire?	
52. Does the child try to minimize or hide their gender?	
53. Does the child ignore their own wetting/soiling?	
54. Does the child play with or smear their feces?	
55. Does the child have problems remembering facts about the trauma?	
56. Does the child often mix up the fact sequence about current events?	

57. Does the child accuse others of things that they could not possibly have done?	
58. Does the child accuse others of doing things that were done by people associated with the trauma?	
59. Does the child seem to be apathetic, uninterested, bored?	
60. Does the child express low self-esteem?	
61. Does the child choose to socially isolate?	
62. Does the child have trouble engaging in cooperative play?	
63. Does the child become oppositional and defensive when given simple directives?	
64. Does the child set themselves up for rejection in relationships?	
65. Does the child have frequent friend changes?	
66. Does the child approach strangers with far too great familiarity?	
67. Does it feel as if the child is not "connecting" with you?	
68. Does the child seem to jump to conclusions or misinterpret what you say?	
69. Do other children shun the child?	
70. Does the child damage or destroy particular items in a methodical and predictable way?	
71. Does the child seem to misbehave just to get your attention?	
72. Does the child get into frequent arguments with siblings or peers?	
73. Does the child engage in "stubborn" behaviors?	
74. Does the child have trouble getting or staying asleep?	
75. Does the child have trouble assessing danger?	
76. Does the child have bouts of explosive anger and rage?	
77. Does the child seem to have focus and attention problems?	
78. Does the child masturbate publicly or excessively?	
79. Does the child complain about being tired?	
80. Does the child engage in risky activities or play?	
81. Does the child express despair?	
82. Does the child view the world as an excessively dangerous place?	
83. Does the child demonstrate mistrust of others?	
84. Is the child very cautious around other people? (male, female, other children?)	
85. Does the child talk about having secrets?	
86. Is the child generally secretive?	
87. Does the child have problems comforting themselves when upset?	
88. Does the child self-comfort in odd ways? (head banging, masturbation, etc.)	

89. Does the child seem to have too much knowledge about sex for their age?	
90. Does the child question every directive or request, no matter how simple?	
91. Does the child verbalize or appear anxious that they will be abandoned?	
92. Is the child excessively physically clingy?	
93. Does the child insist on knowing where significant others are located at all times?	
94. Does the child verbalize that they are to blame for the trauma?	
95. Does the child show signs of low ego cohesion when upset?	
96. Does the child ever appear to be panicked?	
97. Does the child engage in any self-harm behaviors?	
98. Does the child seem to be overly attached or obsessed with a person associated with the trauma?	
99. Does the child frequently express shame or guilt?	
100. Does the child present to others as vulnerable?	
101. Does the child present to others as an inviting victim?	
102. Does the child have behavioral changes following contact with particular people?	

Scoring Summaries

Child's Name:_____   Date:_____

Range	Sub-scale	D	FN	NI	FI
Items 1-27	Allostatic process and load (27)				
Items 28-44	Re-experience (17)				
Items 45-60	Avoidance, numbing & detachment (16)				
Items 61-72	Personal relationships (12)				
Items 73-90	Psychological alterations (18)				
Items 91-102	Self structure (12)				
	Totals				

Date:_____

Range	Sub-scale	D	FN	NI	FI
Items 1-27	Allostatic process and load (27)				
Items 28-44	Re-experience (17)				
Items 45-60	Avoidance, numbing & detachment (16)				
Items 61-72	Personal relationships (12)				
Items 73-90	Psychological alterations (18)				
Items 91-102	Self structure (12)				
	Totals				

Date:_____

Range	Sub-scale	D	FN	NI	FI
Items 1-27	Allostatic process and load (27)				
Items 28-44	Re-experience (17)				
Items 45-60	Avoidance, numbing & detachment (16)				
Items 61-72	Personal relationships (12)				
Items 73-90	Psychological alterations (18)				
Items 91-102	Self structure (12)				
	Totals				

Appendix B: Handouts for Caregivers

[QT2] Caregiver's Instructions for Enuresis

1. If the child does not wet during the daytime, DO NOT put the child into nighttime diapers or pull-ups. As tempting as this is, this only extends the problem. The child needs to feel wet. The key to the plan below is consistency and methodical, determined, strict adherence to the plan.

2. Consider seeing the child's doctor for a prescription of DDAVP, a medication that can help with wetting.

3. Limit liquids in the evening and have a cutoff time for any drinks. Adjust this backwards by fifteen minutes for each week that the current cutoff time is not working.

4. The last adult to bed (assuming this is later than the child) should wake the child to use the toilet. If you can find out when the wetting usually happens, wake the child thirty minutes prior to use the toilet.

5. If you have a new mattress, leave the heavy plastic wrapper on it that it came with. If it is an older mattress, go to the mattress store and see if they will give you the old cover from a display model. Make sure a fresh set of bed sheets and pajamas are in the child's room so that the child can change their bed (right away, before anything else) if it is wet in the morning. If the child is not all over the bed at night, you can fold an old blanket several times and place it under their bottom, to absorb the urine. Or, you can buy a disposable product called "Chux" in a medical supply store.

6. Have the child wake thirty minutes earlier than usual, and see if the bed is wet: sometimes, you might be able to get them to the toilet if a child voids just prior to their usual wake up time. If he or she is wet, the extra time should be used to have the child shower, change their bed, and place wet sheets in the laundry. This also avoids the "yuck" factor of discovering the wet sheets at the next bedtime.

7. Consider investing in a bedwetting alarm: they range in price from about fifty to over a hundred dollars. For some children, the alarm allows them enough time to stop their flow and get to the toilet, and more importantly, by awakening them, teaches their sleepy heads to wake when they feel the pressure to void.

8. If the child is using sleep medication, consult with the doctor to see if a lower dose may be still effective. Sometimes, the child may be so deeply asleep, they cannot wake enough to use the toilet.

9. Treat the bedwetting as a matter of fact issue; never give consequences for bedwetting. Bedwetting is a problem, but not the child. Remind the child that you want to help them to be comfortable, clean, and healthy. Remind them that you are there to support them in making progress on ending the problem, and the problem may take time to solve.

[QT3] Caregiver's Instructions for Encopresis

1. If the child does not soil during the daytime, DO NOT put the child into nighttime diapers or pull-ups. As tempting as this is, this only extends the problem. The child needs to feel the sensation of feces in their underwear. The key to the plan below is consistency and methodical, determined, strict adherence to the plan.

2. Consider seeing the child's doctor for and exam to rule out any physical problems. The doctor may prescribe a stool softener if the child's stools are very dry; the doctor may even prescribe a suppository to induce a bowel movement. But before this is done, the doctor needs to know if the child has been sexually abused anally.

3. If soiling is happening at night, the child should be directed to try to have a bowel movement right after dinner, and right after evening snack. If the child resists this, set up a reward system with your clinician to motivate the child to cooperate. Remember to make the whole process, if not fun, low stress.

4. The last adult to bed (assuming this is later than the child) should check the child to see if they have had a bowel movement in their sleep. A schedule should be made to do this check every hour to ascertain if there is a predictable time that the child moves their bowels.

5. If a predictable time is discovered, the child should be woken up thirty minutes before, and directed to use the potty.

6. If you have new mattress, leave the heavy plastic wrapper on it that it came with. If it is an older mattress, ask the mattress store salesperson if they will give you the old cover from a display model. Make sure a fresh set of bed sheets and pajamas are in the child's room so that the child can change their bed (right away, before anything else) if it is soiled in the morning.

7. Have the child wake thirty minutes earlier than usual, and see if they or their bed is soiled: sometimes, you might be able to get them to the toilet if a child has a bowel movement just prior to their usual wake up time. This is especially important if the child also manipulates their feces. If he or she is soiled, the extra time should be used to have the child shower, change the bed, and place wet sheets in the laundry. This also avoids the "yuck" factor of discovering the wet sheets at the next bed-time.

8. Consider investing in removal of carpets to be replaced by linoleum for the floors, and a highly washable, thick paint for the walls of the bedroom if the child engages in smearing.

9. If the child is using sleep medication, consult with the doctor to see if a lower dose may be still effective. Sometimes, the child may be so deeply asleep, they cannot wake enough to use the toilet.

10. Treat the soiling as a matter of fact issue; never give consequences for soiling. Soiling is a problem, but not the child. Remind the child that you want to help them to be comfortable, clean, and healthy. Remind them that you are there to support them in making progress on ending the problem, and the problem may take time to solve.

Appendix "C" - Quick Teach Sheets

What follows are the 'Quick Tech' sheets that I mentioned earlier in the text. I have had great success with them, with many dozens of them being handed out at seminars, and to just about every adult who may have some interaction with the children I work with.

The Quick Teach sheets are intended as handouts to others who have some kind of association or care for the child. Other professionals, like teachers, ministers, judges, and case managers are often quite busy and do not have time for an extended conversation, but may be able to make use of quick, readable articles such as these. They are also great for foster parents, in order to give them a reference to go back to following education by the clinician. Feel free to copy them and use them as educational tools in your work.

[QT4] Complex PTSD in Children

The diagnosis of PTSD is very specific, and has very specific rules for diagnosis. The child must have experienced one particular event that produced symptoms from a list of three particular categories. The diagnosis and rules for diagnosing it is largely based on work done in the 1960s and 1970s on soldiers coming back from Viet Nam.

Since that time, there has been much more learned about stress disorders, and mental health professionals now speak in terms of "complex PTSD." This means that the person suffering from PTSD may have more than one event that caused their stress disorder, and multiple and complex behaviors associated with it. Some mental health professionals speak about "rolling stress." What is meant by this is that some children who have lived in very chaotic and inconsistent environments develop many of the same symptoms that are seen in classic PTSD.

The idea of many traumatic events happening to a child is not news to those who work with children in foster care. In most cases, these children have some kind of mental health disorder, and have many signs of high stress and reactivity resulting in acting out behaviors. In cases where the child has been physically or sexually abused, there have been multiple events of this type that have contributed to the behavioral symptom the child demonstrates.

Since the diagnosis for PTSD was based largely on adults, and adults coming home from battle conditions in war, the symptoms and behavioral signs were shaped around the adult's experience. Once veterans began to be diagnosed, mental health professionals began to notice that other people who had experienced traumatic events (such as rapes, natural disasters, etc.) also had similar symptoms as did the veterans. It was only natural and logical that victims of other traumas received a closer looking over for PTSD signs.

Though children who have PTSD do demonstrate classic signs of the disorder, they also can express these signs in ways that are specific to children and are not seen in adults. As such, children who are diagnosed with PTSD may have had many other diagnoses and treatments for those diagnoses before they were discovered to really have PTSD.

The three classic symptom clusters in the diagnosis of PTSD are:
- Re-experiencing symptoms.
- Avoidance, numbing, and detachment symptoms.
- Affect dysregulation and arousal dysregulation.

Three other symptoms clusters that many mental health professionals recognize as important to PTSD are:

- Psychological alteration symptoms.
- Relational damage symptoms.
- Ego structure damage symptoms.

[QT5] False Accusations: Confabulation in Children with PTSD

Children who have a diagnosis of PTSD as a result of interpersonal abuse trauma have a long treatment road to recovery. One aspect of this recovery is their ability to process the abuse history in a positive manner that allows them to move beyond the terrifying memories of abuse. This processing may take from many months to many years, and along the way the child may develop some behavioral signs that are difficult, if not mistaken ways of working through their history of abuse.

One of the things that these children tend to do is to make false accusations at some point during their treatment, and sometimes several times during treatment. These false accusations can be made towards anyone the child knows, but most often, they are made towards people that the child is very comfortable with, such as foster parents, teachers, or counselors.

There are several reasons why children make the false accusations. Some of these include the fact that the child has become comfortable with certain adults. The child comes to consider the adult a 'safe' person to work through their abuse history with. When the child accuses the innocent adult, this may be a 'transference' effect. Transference is when the child 'transfers' the angry feelings towards their abuser to a safe person to express them with. This of course, causes havoc for the innocent adult. Nonetheless, all reports by the child of abuse must be followed up upon and investigated. The point is for others to understand that the accusation very well could be false. Much research demonstrates that children do misrepresent the truth about abuse, and this applies both to children who have never been abused, and those who have.

The other reason for false accusation is that all children want to please adults, and are at times anxious when being questioned by adults. If the child has a strong desire to please the adult, and the child perceives that their answer was not satisfying to the adult, they may in fact give a different answer that indicates abuse. It does not take much for the child to perceive that the answer that they have given did not satisfy the adult who is questioning them, and children are generally bright enough to 'read between the lines' to understand that the adult may be suspecting abuse. The secondary reason for this confabulating effect is that many abused children have learned in the past to use confabulation to avoid more abuse from their abuser. This is learned self preservation and victim behavior.

Children who have been physically or sexually abused may also often make reports of 'phantom pain' due to past abuse. The injury being reported could be an injury experienced months or even years before. They may point our very small injuries that are normal for all children, and express an account of how they got the injury that is clearly abusive. The problem is, they may be describing an event of abuse that happened long ago, and has nothing to do with the small scratch on their arm. The ignorance of the adult listener concerning these effects could lead the adult to believe that abuse has taken place in the past twenty four hours. These effects, like the others mentioned, can be stimulated by all kinds of cues and triggers in the child's environment. Essentially, something in the child's environment may stimulate a bad memory. Once the bad memory is activated, the child may begin to experience strong emotions, and re-experience physical symptoms of the abuse that occurred in the past.

It is important that adults speaking with children who have been abused understand that these things will likely happen as part of the child's healing process. They also need to realize that the child is not lying in the classical sense, but is confabulating based upon the symptoms of their PTSD. Further, adults should recognize that they can unconsciously lead the child to make false accusations. Even a facial expression or tone of voice can press a PTSD child to make a confabulation. When an untrained adult suspects that a child has been abused, they should limit their questions, and refer the child to a professional who specializes in such abuse cases.

[QT6] Encopresis and Enuresis in Stress Disordered Children

Children with stress disorders (Acute Stress or Post Traumatic Stress) often suffer from encopresis or enuresis, or both. Encopresis is typically a consistent soiling of feces in the clothing, despite previously known toilet learning. This sometimes is just a small amount, or it can be large amounts of feces. In some children with a stress disorder, they may also "play with" the feces, smearing themselves or the environment with feces. Encopresis may be accompanied by enuresis, or wetting. The wetting may occur both at night and during the daytime in otherwise toilet competent children. Some children simply wet the bed or themselves, while others may void in inappropriate place when a toilet is readily available.

The reasons for both problems can be multi-layered. There may be more than one source for any particular child's toileting issues. Some children may have not had adequate toilet learning or scheduling, and may have a physical disruption of the normal bowel process due to consistent withholding of feces. The child may have begun to withhold due to having a painful bowel movement, or from having gotten into trouble with an adult when they had a genuine accident. In essence, they may have developed a poor bowel habit. In addition, a child may have experienced emotional and physical regression following a single, very frightening trauma. In this case, the toileting problem may resolve itself once the child begins to feel secure again.

The effect of losing control of one's bladder and bowels when deeply frightened is well-documented. A child who has been repeatedly frightened may develop an automatic, uncontrollable elimination whenever they begin to be frightened about *anything*, and by *anyone*, not just the perpetrator of their traumatic abuse. They may even have the effect when they have had an intrusive memory or nightmare about their original trauma. This effect is not just due to a muscular release, but also likely due to intense chemical changes in the child's body when they are frightened.

In other cases, there may be the additional layer of the child's anger. All cultural myths to the contrary, children do not have much control over the adults in their lives. When a child becomes very angry at an adult, they have few options to "get back" at the adult. In most cases, these children do not have adequate learning in how to positively express negative emotions. They also do not have good role models on how to express anger. Nothing quite strikes back at an adult that the child is angry at than soiling themselves and smearing the results on the walls.

Still yet another possibility for the behaviors is that the child has used them as a defense against sexual abuse. Again, the feces and urine may be a very effective way for the child to keep a sexual perpetrator away.

Untangling the source(s) for the behaviors is thus not an easy task, and it takes time, close observations and tracking of behaviors, and above all, patience. It is important for those treating stress disordered children with encopretic and enuretic problems to understand that the child is not engaging in the behaviors to get *you* angry per-se. The behaviors are a reaction to old history and traumatic events in their lives.

In most cases, all of the "practical" advice that is given on these issues, while it may ease the problem, does not solve it. The real solution lies in helping the child to gain improved, age appropriate ego strength and a healthy level of differentiation. In doing this, the child is able to adequately face and process the horrible traumas that they have endured, and in turn, find more positive and effective ways to express their pain, fear, and anger.

[QT7] Fostering a Sexually Abused Child

Children who have been abused sexually have specific needs in foster care. Foster parents need to understand several aspects of how sexually abused children express symptoms. Though sexually abused children present some challenges that other children who have not been sexually abused do not present, they are still just children in need of love, affection, care, and guidance.

The first thing that foster parents need to understand is the child's diagnosis. Often, children who have been sexually abused will have a diagnosis of Post Traumatic Stress Disorder. If this is the case, the foster parent should read up on this disorder in the other articles dedicated to PTSD in children in this series. Other children may not have a PTSD diagnosis, but have some other diagnosis such as Oppositional Defiant Disorder or Reactive Attachment Disorder.

Abused children express their issues of sexual abuse in a variety of ways. Some children have a cluster of behaviors that has been termed: "Child Sexual Abuse Accommodation Syndrome (CSAAS)." The CSAAS was developed in 1983 by Dr. Roland Summit as a descriptor of signs seen frequently in sexually abused children. This is a description of behaviors that many, but not all, sexually abuse children demonstrate. These behaviors include:

- Secrecy about the abuse, reluctance to speak about it due to possible threats by the perpetrator.
- Emotional helplessness to resist or complain about the original abuse, or subsequent re-victimization by other perpetrators.
- Entrapment and accommodation, in that the child feels that there is no way to escape the abuse, so they learn to cope with it and adapt. The child's resolve to tell also may "fold" in the presence of the perpetrator or other persons associated with the perpetrator.
- Delayed, conflicted, and unconvincing disclosure of the abuse. This disclosure may seem exaggerated, inconsistent in detail, or simply vague.

The child may "backpedal" or recant their allegations to restore the family structure, or to emotionally calm a parent, family member, or the perpetrator.

There are other behavioral difficulties that can occur in sexually abused children. They may have behaviors that are sexually pre-occupied: they may use vulgar language, or speak about sexual issues with other children. Some children may masturbate excessively, to self-comfort, or masturbate in public. They may behave or try to dress in ways that are seductive or amorous. Some children may make attempts at sexual contact with other children or adults. On the other hand, some children who are sexually abused may try to minimize their gender, and be highly concerned about their privacy, and reject physical affection..

Children who have behaviors that are sexually precocious need to be given firm, but non-punitive guidance about appropriateness and boundaries. For some of these children, it is not wise to allow them out of your sight for long periods of time when they are interacting with other, especially younger children. Though in most cases, no genuinely dangerous activities will take place, it is very important for the child not to engage in behaviors that can become a pattern of sexualized, clandestine and manipulative sexualized behaviors with other children.

There will be occasions when a sexually abused child will begin to "tell" a foster parent about a specific event of sexual abuse. When this occurs, the foster parent needs to keep in mind two basic things: accurate recording of what the child said, and avoiding certain types of questioning that could make the information gained essentially worthless in protecting the child. While it is therapeutically desirable for the child to verbalize about their abuse, foster parents should realize that there is a very strict set of guidelines about what can be accepted as evidence by child protection workers, and is acceptable in court as testimony. When a child's accounts are tainted by the wrong methods of questioning, they are likely to be discarded by the legal system. Though there is only a small chance that a foster parent would ever be called to court to testify in a situation where a foster child reveals sexual abuse details, foster parents should be prepared.

Foster parents needs to know that children often reveal information about abuse in one of two ways: either they blurt it out once they gain trust in an adult, or they accidentally speak about it. When possible, a foster parent should seek help from the child's therapist in processing such material; there are many complexities to communications with children about sexual abuse issues. There are even many professional therapists who make common mistakes in these conversations with children. Research shows that children's memories and accountings of sexual abuse can be quite accurate, and they generally do not make up stories about the abuse... except when the wrong approach to questioning is used by well meaning adults. But of course, the child may not be willing to speak to the therapist if there is a wait. In these cases, the foster parent should keep these guidelines in mind:

- Remember that children want to please adults; the child may give an embellished answer to satisfy you.
- Remember that you are a big person, and the child is small; this can be intimidating, and the child may give a made up answer just to get you to back off.

- Never "lead" a child with questions. Here are some examples of subtle, leading questions:
- "If someone has done sexual things with you, did they do (whatever)?" Or, perhaps more commonly: "Has anyone ever touched you inappropriately?"
- Never suggest an emotion or content to the child that the child has not expressed. For example: "I'll bet that it would be frightening if an adult tried to put their hands down your pants."
- If you repeat a question, the child may assume that their first answer was not 'good enough', and then try to embellish the answer to satisfy you.
- Never ask "trap questions": "Did this person do (this) or (that)? This leaves the child only two answers, either one being a positive statement about abuse.
- Be aware that if the child begins to talk about sexual abuse, and you already know the child has been sexually abused, you may have a bias about who the perpetrator is, and what was done.

The following are better strategies if the child begins to reveal to you:

- Stay calm; hide your anxieties, fears, or anger towards the perpetrator.
- Use small encouragements to encourage the child to speak, such as: "Hmmm..." or "I see". You can also nod your head and keep eye contact and appropriate physical proximity.
- If you *must* ask a question, just say: "I don't quite understand, can you tell me more?"
- If you want to add emotional support, simply reflect an emotion that the child is giving, or, you can ask the child how they felt at the time, or how they now feel.
- If the child makes any statements that the abuse was somehow their fault, immediately correct this, telling the child sexual (or any) abuse is never a child's fault.
- Reassure the child that you will keep them safe. Tell the child that it might be necessary for someone else to talk to the child about their statements (you need not say who just now) so that the child can remain safe, and that you will be with them when they do.
- Report the conversation as soon as possible to the child's other treatment staff, and make a child abuse report if indicated.

[QT8] How Acute Stress and PTSD Behavioral Signs May Be Confused With Normal Child Behaviors

Often, children with Acute Stress Disorder or Post Traumatic Stress Disorder have one or more diagnoses behind them before they are accurately diagnosed with a stress disorder. Many caregivers see the behavioral signs that the child is demonstrating and come to the conclusion that the child may be ADHD, very oppositional, or simply under disciplined. Though many of the behavioral signs of stress disorders are common to other disorders, when the total inventory of signs is viewed, along with any known traumatic history, the diagnosis becomes quite evident.

In cases where the child is living with their biological parent(s), and there is an intergenerational history of domestic abuse, addiction, or child abuse, the adults may either be in denial of the possibility of a stress disorder (or an event that has caused it), or they have become numb themselves and do not have the perspective to recognize the behaviors as abnormal.

Below is an overview of how each of the six behavioral sign clusters may be confused with normal childhood behaviors.

Allostatic behavioral signs

These behavioral signs at first may be mistaken for hyperactivity or simple childhood excitement, but these signs tend to be much more intense, and not in relation to the situation around the child. The child at times seems to become very agitated, anxious, aggressive, overly shy, or very fearful for no real apparent reason, or there appears to be an overreaction to some event or situation. The child may become very silly or overly familiar with strangers. The child often has a very hard time calming down. There may be problems with sleep: getting to sleep, staying asleep, and nightmares. The child may startle very easily, and may be overly clingy towards caregivers. The child's appetite and bowel-bladder habits may be affected. There is often an increase in toileting accidents, intentional toileting in closets, corners, etc. The child may actually manipulate or play with their own or animal feces. There may be regressions, slow, or stalled potty learning in younger children. Children may also express a sudden change of affect: their expression may become flat, pupils may dilate, and the child will look as if they are daydreaming, or "off in their own world".

These behavioral signs can occur at any time the child is "triggered" by someone, some thing, or some location in their environment. The number and kind of triggers can be difficult to ascertain, especially in younger children. When there is a dramatic increase in agitation following contact with a person who is a trigger, this is often confused with the child being upset, sad, or disappointed that they are no longer in the person's presence or care. The key differences between a triggered PTSD episode and the child simply missing the person is that the signs are much more intense, of longer duration, and include hours if not days of severe and consistent misbehavior as well as an increase of the other five sign clusters.

Re-experiencing

These behavioral signs may be confused with a child's normal play; children may engage in violent play or re-enactments of traumatic events in their lives with action figures or dolls. The child may also become oppositional over small issues; they may seem to need to be in control of every situation to feel comfortable. This may be confused with "stubbornness" and "being contrary". The difference is that when an average child is pressed, they will give in; when a stressed child is pressed, their agitation increases to the point of getting out of control. Children who have been sexually abused may engage in more frequent and public masturbation or simulated sex acts. They may also engage in odd behaviors, such as stuffing toilet paper or other objects in their pants. They may use explicitly sexual language, or have precocious knowledge about sex. Nightmares are a form of re-experiencing. When a child is triggered and becomes physically agitated, their body is essentially doing the same thing it did when they were experiencing the trauma. When the child is highly agitated and their expression becomes very flat, or their eyes "glaze over", they are likely re-experiencing the trauma.

Avoidance, numbing and detachment

This behavioral cluster can be confused with a child trying to avoid responsibilities, being stubborn, or being angry at family members. The child may actively avoid certain people, places, or items. They may seem to have "forgotten all about" the traumatic event that took place, or their recent acting out/stress episode. The child may not respond to every day injuries like other children; they may easily shake off scrapes and bumps without tears or any reaction at all. On the other hand, they may become very upset and over reactive to very slight injuries. The child may seem to "bully" other children by simply ignoring the other child and "plowing on through". The child may actually physically attack another child with pinching, biting, hitting, or strangling. This may be confused with sibling rivalry or peer disagreements, but the marker is the frequency and intensity of the behaviors. They may seem to have little empathy for other people who are injured or have their feelings hurt. In most stress disordered children, there is often a lack of the ability to self comfort. In play, it can also be seen that the child has not formed much attachment to any one toy; the child may not have a cuddle toy, for example.

Psychological alterations

These behavioral signs may be confused with a child who is "spoiled". The child may continue to try to sleep in the caregiver's bed, they may show regressed developmental behaviors, such as daytime wetting, using "baby talk", a desire to use a pacifier or bottle ,or becoming very clingy to the caregiver. The child may exhibit memory problems or confabulate wild stories or fantasies that are considerably more detailed or odd than the average child's "active imagination". The child may become hypervigilant; they may be very watchful and seem anxious, or fearful of being abandoned. The child may be very impulsive, and engage in risky play without apparent understanding of the danger. The child may either have gained a very hostile and negative attitude towards the world, or they present themselves to others as very vulnerable, and then get taken advantage of or are re-victimized.

Relational problems

This set of behavioral signs may be confused with an over shyness, or a child who "has not had the right discipline", or is "full of themselves". The child may have trouble trusting others, may be secretive and very guarded. The child may have problems making and keeping friends. They may "try too hard" to be friendly or to fit in. The child may become very bossy and parentified. There may physical boundary problems in the way the child relates to others, such as standing too close, touching too freely or too soon in a relationship. The child may touch others inappropriately, such as tickling or sexualized touching. The child may seem to crave help, care, and affection, but when it is given, push the helper away. These children will often be quickly identified as behavior problems when they start school.

Ego structure

These behavioral signs may be confused with a child who is simply "down" or depressed. The child may seem to be very emotionally fragile and "fall apart" easily. They may verbalize low self-esteem, or blame themselves for the bad things that have happened to them. The child may alternate from being very oppositional to being excessively cooperative and easily led. There may be periods of time where the child retreats into extraordinarily detailed fantasy. They may even have their own secret language have different names for themselves.

Essentially, the markers for a child with a stress disorder as opposed to normal childhood behaviors becomes: the presence of all six clusters of behavioral signs, the intensity of the signs above average childhood behaviors, and the frequency at which they occur.

[QT9] Stress Signs in Children with PTSD

Re-experiencing

- Intrusive dreams, nightmares
- Daytime intrusive memories
- Physical agitation
- Anger/rage
- Severe upsets over apparently small issues
- Enuresis, encopresis
- Play reenactments
- Hiding
- Physically aggressive, combative
- Complaints about wounds, pain, boo-boos that you cannot see present
- Talking about or relating details about the trauma

Avoidance, numbing, detachment

- Avoids discussing trauma or people associated
- Lack of empathy or sympathy
- Bullying/hurting others with no remorse
- Lack of connectivity with others
- Ignoring others' feelings, statements, directives, conversation, assistance
- Emotional numbing
- Physical numbing
- Self-harm, disregard for danger or injuries
- Lacks age appropriate play or activity
- Cruelty to animals
- Lack of focus
- Overly submissive
- Cannot describe their emotions
- Consistently misinterpreting what others are saying
- Socially isolating
- Can't remember obvious time lines or events

Increased arousal

- Physical agitation, aggression
- Trashing their toys, clothes, room
- Door slamming
- Screaming
- Foul language not usually heard
- Hyperactive
- Hyper reactive
- Jumpy, easily startles
- Hypervigilant
- Fight or flight behaviors
- Helpless
- Frozen
- Glassy eyes, dilated pupils, zombie like
- Lack of focus/attention
- Oppositional, defensive
- Sexualized behaviors
- Argumentative
- Hiding behaviors (food, self, soiled clothes)
- Easily brought to tears
- Rushing through work, schoolwork, doing a poor job
- Cannot seem to calm down for hours upon hours, or even days

Psychological alterations

- Age regressed behaviors
- Heightened vulnerability
- Emotional cycling
- Memory difficulties
- Chronic fatigue, physical complaints
- Risk taking
- Heightened impulsivity
- Statements of despair
- Can't seem to comfort self

Relational

- Mistrust
- Heightened accusations against others
- Secretive
- Guarded
- Self defeating interactions
- Child like or precocious
- Worried about being abandoned or left behind
- Increased boundary problems
- Inconsistent approach, friendliness, affect in relating
- Seems to try too hard to fit in
- Makes complaints about being excluded by others
- Argumentative for no apparent reason
- Bossy, parentified
- Clingy, seeking attention
- Excessive seeking out of nurturing/comfort
- "Push-pull" feeling of intimacy and care
- Refusal of assistance, help, care, affection.
- Calls older relatives by first name

Ego structure

- Attributes traumatic events to their fault
- Self-harm verbalizations
- Seems to "fall apart" very easily
- Shame, guilt. Low self-esteem statements
- Has multiple names either given to them or for themselves
- Alteration between very stubborn and excessively vulnerable

[QT10] Recognizing Stress in Children

We all have been in a situation where a child in our care is highly stressed. It is usually quite obvious: they are having a tantrum! But tantrum behavior is the end result of a series of signs. It is important to be able spot the more subtle signs and then make interventions before the child gets to the state of a full blown tantrum.

The first thing to look for is the amount of simulation that the child has recently had or is currently having. Extreme stimulation can pour chemicals into the child's bloodstream and create stress behaviors. The fancy term for this is "allostatic load". As the body responds to the new levels of stimulation, predictable behaviors begin to emerge. For a child, "stimulation" can be such things as: getting too excited around peers at a party, school tests, being pressured to comply with directives, or contact with particular people.

If you think of a glass of water, everyone has a particular capacity for stress before the glass "overflows". The overflow is the stress signs. Most children have a set of coping strategies that they have learned from a very young age, and can maintain good behavior even when stressed. Other children, who have not had this kind of early learning, or come from very difficult and stressed families, often are very reactive to even minor stressors. This is a good sign to watch for: if the child becomes hyper-reactive to minor stressors.

Stress also can show up as an increased anxiety. The child may appear to be hyperactive, and seems to become very picky or obsessed about minor things. They may find it very hard to calm down for any length of time, even with your help to do so. Adults may find themselves telling the child over and over again to "relax", or "calm down".

Other signs to look for include a general pattern of fight-or-flight. This can mean literally fighting physically or verbally, or running away. But it may not be so dramatic a flight; a child may begin to isolate or withdraw from the family and peers, or they may begin to rush through their schoolwork or chores, not completing or making many mistakes. They also may begin to stop engaging in preferred activities as a form of flight. Some younger children may hide in closets or under their beds. As the adult, you may feel the "space" between you and the child begin to open up; like the child is drifting away in the relationship. Children may become contentious and escalate sibling rivalries as a form of "fight".

More subtly, children often have a lowered capacity for internal monitoring when very stressed. This means that they have a hard time knowing and expressing what they feel. When an adult recognizes that the child is having difficulty and asks the child about it, the child will have a tough time explaining what is going on. Many children will simply state: "I don't know", or not give a response at all. Unfortunately, if the adult does not ask the question in the right way, the child will likely feel that they are being corrected (read: persecuted).

Also, children who are under stress will quite often have very altered and distorted thinking. When they try to express themselves, it may be hard to follow. Their logic is often flawed, and they will reject any logic presented to them. They also may have a hard time in relating the proper chronology of a particular event.

The earlier the signs of stress in a child are recognized, the earlier an intervention can be made to help avoid a full blown tantrum, or lower the intensity of the oncoming behaviors.

[QT11] Responding to a Highly Stressed Child

When a child in our care is highly stressed, so are we. This is a fact, and one that is important to an effective response to help the child. We need to keep in mind that strong emotions are often contagious. While we will always have some level of stress when dealing with a stressed child, we must guard against "catching" the full brunt of their stress. Often, children, because they know us, will be very skilled in attacking us verbally when they are stressed. The biggest mistake we can make is to *personalize this material.*

A second mistake that most adults make when addressing a highly stressed child is to begin to increase the pressure on the child to comply. From experience, this hardly ever works. It usually just escalates the situation further. So what to do?

Fortunately, there are skills that you can build to help children in your care to lower their stress. The first is to recognize that lowering a highly stressed child takes space and time. Every child and every situation has its own timetable for de-escalation. You *cannot rush* the process. The space where you find yourself with the child is also important. If possible, lower the stimulation in the space; turn off televisions, radios, etc. Direct other people that are not needed in the room to leave. If the child is in a space not appropriate for de-escalation, try to gently encourage the child to let you guide them to another, less public area.

Your next tool is your tone of voice. In giving directives, it should be firm, confident, and compassionate. It should be used at normal volume. In engagement about the issue at hand or what is stressing the child, you voice should be what I call a "Mr. Rogers" voice. This is calm, gentle, and nurturing. Many people become uncomfortable with this approach, thinking that the intention is to "coddle" the child; it is not. You can maintain a calm, gentle, and nurturing tone while continuing to be firm and unyielding to your behavioral standards and expectations.

It is important when approaching a stressed child to first ask permission to get physically close to them, or at least tell them that you are going to move closer. This demonstrates respect for their emotional state; it is also wise to do from the standpoint that the child may feel threatened by your sudden move closer to them. If you ask, and they allow it, you might sit close enough to them for physical contact (arm to arm). If they also allow, put an arm around them, or pat their back. If you can get to this point, the child will often calm noticeably, and may even begin to cry instead of tantrum.

Your goal is to help the child calm with your voice and reassuring presence. At times, stressed children may try to harm themselves. If they do, you must tell them in the same calm, nurturing voice, that you will not let them do that. If they lash out at you physically, simply move away, out of range. If they head bang or begin to hit themselves, put a pillow, stuffed animal, or your hand between.

Once the child calms a bit, you might begin to ask them (not press them) what they are thinking and feeling. The idea is to get them to *process* the source of their stress in a positive and effective manner. Remember to give them time enough to calm enough to do this. If they at first refuse, fall back to your kind, firm, nurturing, and try to get them to process a bit later. You can also give honest reassurances that things will get better. Do not make any promises that you cannot keep. *Never* offer any kind of bribes for the child to stop their upset. End the event with a strong suggestion that when they are upset again, they can come to you and *process* their concerns and feelings, rather than become over stressed and tantrum. Follow this up with a hug and assertive statement that you care very much for them.

[QT12] Response Particulars to a Stress Disordered Child

Often, in the treatment of children with diagnosed stress disorders, the treatment approach of the adult (*what* the adult does, and *how* the adult responds) is counter-intuitive to how we might ordinarily respond to an acting out child.

The following response particulars will be presented this way: the *behavior* the child is engaging in, the *adult response*, and then the reason for that response.

Building stress: Once we become aware that a child is stressed ,we need to respond appropriately. If we do not, the child will likely escalate in their behaviors. Most adults can spot when a child is becoming stressed out. Generally, the child with stress disorder will have much more subtle signs over a longer period of time. Adults may need to become much more observant of children who have diagnosed stress disorders. One way to understand the stressed child is to think of a glass of water: we all have some stress in our "glass". A child with stress disorder has a glass that is nearly always full. When enough stress is collected, the glass will overflow with symptoms (behaviors). If signs of stress are spotted early and responded to properly, there can be very good results in treatment.

Cues and triggers: Adults in contact with a child who has a stress disorder diagnosis need to learn about and become sensitive to the child's cue and trigger behaviors. These can be very dramatic, or they can be very subtle and hard to see. If adults do not attend to this important and basic aspect of the child's treatment, the child's healing will be delayed, or even halted entirely.

A stressed child's behaviors come out of cues and triggers. A cue is something in the child's environment that reminds them (often unconsciously) of something related to their trauma event that triggers a stress reaction. A cue can be an item, a smell, a taste, a noise, a tone of voice, a physical gesture, or even just a thought. There can be hundreds of cues for someone with a stress disorder, and other people cannot do much about avoiding them. Sometimes, a particular few cues and known triggers are revealed, and then these can be avoided, especially by those adults treating the child. Cue and trigger behaviors for a child may include such things as increased distractibility, finger nail chewing, glassy eyed stare, apparent ignoring of adults or peers, combativeness, or physical intrusions. Many other cue and trigger behaviors follow below.

Stress Break: Constructing a routine "stress break" for the child can be very effective in heading off full blown stress episodes. It also supports the treatment objective of helping the child to recognize their own stress levels and learning how to self calm. The break can be as simple as allowing or directing the child to engage in a behavior that is known to be calming to them. This could be cuddling a stuffed animal, listening to music, reading a story book, doing prescribed breathing exercises, or playing with a toy. In the classroom, a "secret signal" can be arranged between the adult and the child, so that the child may access (or the teacher direct) a stress break quickly, with little distraction in the classroom. Many adults feel that such breaks are indulgent to the child. They see the acting out behaviors in the context of either defiance or a spoiled child. Nothing could be further from the child's reality. These adults are not understanding the intensity and anguish of internal distress that the child is undergoing. Essentially, when a child has been cued and triggered into a stress episode, their bodies and minds are reacting the same exact way that they did when their original trauma was taking place (read: flood, earthquake, fire, rape, physical abuse, sexual abuse, food deprivation). Once this is understood, any adult should be able to be compassionate and begin to follow a treatment plan that is designed to help the child avoid escalations of this highly painful state.

Defiance or general acting out: Use a normal voice tone devoid of pressure and inflection. Try to keep your voice as neutral as possible, but firm. Make your directive brief and to the point. You may repeat the directive once more, but do not keep repeating or elaborating. You may choose to direct the child to take a "stress break." Following your initial presentation, turn away from the child and give them opportunity to self calm, or comply with directive to take a stress break. (See "*stress break*"). You are trying to avoid adding any extra stress or pressure to the child than is absolutely necessary. Most adults add more pressure by raising their voices or making threats to get an oppositional child to respond. With stress disordered children, this only increases their resistance to us, and will likely trigger a full blown stress episode.

Tears, pouting, crying: First, use all of the suggestions above. Try not to react to the tears , pouting, or crying. Treat the upset with matter of fact recognition of their distress. ("I can see that you are upset"). You might offer a choice to the child, and identify the choice that you think is the better one. If the child is expressing tears in an overreaction, you may also say to the effect: "There is no reason to be crying right now....(give directive)." Do not over elaborate or engage in debate with the child. Turn away from the child and allow them time to either self calm or take a stress break. You are trying to communicate to the child that while you can see that they are distressed, they need to follow your directions Your calm voice and low intensity approach tell them that your directions are not threatening to them. If you would raise your voice or intensity, the child will likely trigger to a full blown stress reaction. Children with stress disorder are easily cued and triggered by adults who react to the child in ways the child is anticipating. When we react to the child in ways that (perhaps a perpetrator) did, the child will escalate.

Demanding, hostile, nasty, oppositional: Use all of the responses that appear in "defiance or general acting out." Using a neutral, non-intense tone of voice, give an immediate directive for a "time out". It is important that this "time out" be immediate, and not "later". It is also important that this "time out" be clearly different from a "stress break". This can be done by making the "time out" a particular chair or place (never the bedroom, or out of an adult's sight). You may also call the "time out" place something like "the naughty chair". When giving your directive to go to time out, be very careful about physically approaching the child; do not make sudden gestures, keep proximity reasonably distant. If you approach, approach slowly. It is important to keep your voice tone normal, because if you raise it, you may trigger a larger reaction. Adults do not have to yell or threaten to be effective in being firm! Once again, we need to respond to the child in a manner that is different than what they may have experienced in the past. A stressed child needs to have immediate penalties for misbehavior because one of the symptoms that they may have is a poor memory. This is an effect of the trauma they have experienced. If we wait until later (as in, "no recess for you today"), they will simply experience the later penalty as cruelty. They may also trigger into a stress reaction when recess time comes around.

When the child balks at a directive or given task: By now, you should have the "neutral, firm tone of voice" idea firmly in mind! Remember to avoid debating with the child. Give a choice when appropriate, and encourage that the child "make a good choice". Give your directive, and repeat it once if needed. Give advisement about the consequence of not following the directive or completing the task. Then, turn away and give the child time to self calm or take a stress break. Follow up within five to ten minutes by repeating the directive. If the child continues to refuse, apply the (immediate) consequence. When a child with stress disorder has a negative behavior, it does not always mean that it is stress related, but it could be. That is why you use the same basic "neutral firm tone" when approaching them. Many adults begin to anticipate that each time a stress disordered child is upset, the child will escalate. In anticipation of this, the adult behavior and approach may change subtlety, become more anxious of a bigger upset. It is important to note that the adult's anxiety and stress can actually trigger the child!

Poor attention and lack of focus, and rushing: Again use your neutral, firm tone of voice to give directives to refocus or slow down. This directive can be repeated, but take a closer look at the child following the second prompt. If the inattention and focus problem continues, prompt the child to take a stress break. Children with stress disorders are often labeled "attention deficit-hyperactive" when they are not. When a child is highly stressed (just like you or me), their attention and focus suffer. Their activity may become scattered and disorganized. Rushing through tasks, such as schoolwork or chores, is very common. This rushing is a form of "flight". These signs are a clear sign of building stress towards a full blown stress episode. If adults do not take note of this and provide needed support, there will likely be acting out behavior in the near future.

Bossy or tattling: Using your neutral, firm tone, remind the child that being the boss or tattling is not their job. If they repeat the behavior, make your statement again, but this time with an advisement about an upcoming consequence ("time out"). Children who are stress disordered have had one or more traumatic events in their lives that they had absolutely no control over. Thus, control becomes an important issue to them. Many children become very bossy, or tattle, or become rigid in the way they want something done (how their sandwich is cut, for example). When they do not feel that they have any control, they may escalate because the situation (lack of control) reminds them of when something bad happened. Whenever possible and appropriate, it is good to give choices to a stress disordered child. It is also very wise to be sure that they know upcoming events and situational changes. When these children are surprised, it can trigger feelings of loss of control, and then acting out behavior.

Helpless/hopeless: This is a situation where you can abandon your "neutral, firm tone"! Now is the time for positive, upbeat, and encouraging directives. State your confidence in the child, cite their strengths, give compliments, and then move on. Give the child added encouragement when they begin to demonstrate work and success. Stress disordered children can get very discouraged and tired of their constant, rollercoaster feelings of stress. Imagine having the feeling you get at the top of the first hill on a rollercoaster two or three dozen times a day! These children often need extra nurturing and encouragement, and this is not indulgent to the child. In some cases, the child may have been very deprived of this kind of support in their past. In any case, a child is a child: they need adult nurturing reassurances, and encouragement.

[QT13] Stress Inoculation for Children through Healthy Differentiation

Stress Inoculation is a process to help victims of Post Traumatic Stress Disorder or Acute Stress Disorder to become less reactive to things that remind them of the bad things that have happened to them. Differentiation is a process of growth in a human being. Healthy differentiation is the individual's ability to be able to be in close intimate contact with another person and not feel anxious or "lose hold" of themselves. When a child has healthy differentiation, they are able to stand up for themselves, are free to make their preferences known, naturally set personal boundaries, have a genuine, unique self identity and good self-esteem. A well differentiated child knows that they can openly disagree with adults in a respectful manner. A child with healthy differentiation is able to manage stress by drawing on a reserve of coping skills. Differentiation gives the child the ability to be assertive, take care of themselves, and get along well with others.

Most children who have stress disorders cannot do these things. Many have stress symptoms due to the family experience that they have endured. These children can have very underdeveloped or weakened self identity. When a child lives in an abusive and often chaotic household, they may be unable to adequately develop along a normal emotional growth curve. The parent(s) or caretaker may have such an overwhelming and overbearing way of dealing with the child that the child becomes "fused" with the adult. The child becomes an extension of the adult, and not a person unto themselves. Often, these children are treated as if they were owned objects instead of cherished people. The child becomes a slave to the adult's desires and whims, and a victim of any destructive lifestyle that the adult leads. The child has no control over anything in their life. If the parent or caretaker is also a perpetrator of abuse on the child, the child will live with a "rolling stress" that never lets up. The child never knows when the adult will be kind and caregiving, or cruel and abusive.

It may seem strange that children who live with parents who have mistreated them by neglect or abuse would become over attached (fused) to the parent. But the child has no choice but to cling to their parent, because that is all they have. The child develops an "automatic reaction" when they are around the parent. At the same time that they are fearful and cautious, they may also demonstrate affection and enthusiasm to please the parent. They know the cost of not being cautious, and the benefits of keeping the parent in a good mood.

Children with such a level of constant stress will oftentimes begin to generalize this reactivity to other adults than their abusive parent or caretaker. Many children who are victims of stress disorders become not only victims in their families, but victims to other perpetrators in the community as well, because when under stress, they "roll over" into submission.

When such a child comes into foster care, the foster parents may notice that the child shows both extreme caution and enthusiasm to please early in their care. This is that generalized reactivity: they are doing the same with you as they did with their parent or caretaker. The child will also begin to try to interact with you at a deeper level the same way they did when they were in their biological family. This may include manipulation, threats, or actual verbal and physical assault. The child will bring with them to your family all of the family illness that was in their family. Any time the child is reminded of the bad times in their family, or of a particular traumatic event in their past, they may have a strong stress reaction.

Anything can be a reminder: an object, a smell, a time of day, bathing, or even a tone of voice. Essentially their little bodies react the same way that they did when the trauma was happening. Their heart rate rises, their blood pressure spikes, they begin to breathe differently, chemicals like adrenaline rush into their bloodstream. They enter into a stress episode that may include rage, violence, soiling themselves, harming themselves, among other behaviors. This automatic process can be reversed. The child can get better.

What Is Stress Inoculation?

The challenge is to "inoculate" them to the stress. Stress Inoculation is just like taking a flu shot to avoid getting a full blown case of the flu. The shot itself may be a bit uncomfortable, makes your arm sore for couple of days, and you may even have some mild flu symptoms. When the virus comes around, the inoculation keeps you from getting it, or if you do, it will be a much milder case.

Caring and effective adults treating a child with a traumatic stress disorder help the child when they find ways to encourage the child to differentiate in a healthy, age normal fashion. Remember that differentiation is the individual's ability to be able to be in close intimate contact with another person (or stressor) and not feel anxious or "lose hold" of themselves.

The goal is to end the automatic physical, emotional, and behavioral reactions. One way to do this is to build and develop the child's ego to withstand stress and build emotional freedom with emotional self regulation. They need to be able to "hold on to themselves" when reminders of their trauma appear before them.

Building the child's ego towards their being more differentiated would include providing the child with firm, very clear, very simple boundaries and limits that are repeated frequently. Make clear that the child, too, has the right to state their boundaries and limits. You may need to help them make such a list of limits and boundaries, such as: "no one can come into my room without knocking", "no one hits in this house", or "no one can touch my private area". It is likely that the child has had only inconsistent, confusing, and violated limits and boundaries in the past. Your limits and boundaries as well as helping them to develop their own limits and boundaries helps the child to feel secure.

Giving a child reasonable choices according to his or her age is also a way to help them build their ego strength. Older children may be invited to decorate their own room, or choose their own clothing purchases. To be able to have some freedom to self govern, even if it is only a choice to have their bath now or after dinner, is an ego building technique.

You cannot give a child who is stress disordered enough positive attention and affection. Most are very hungry for these positive strokes. Acknowledging positive behaviors, celebrating individuality and unique talents, and letting the child know that they are valued are all ego builders that develop healthy differentiation.

When the child was with their biological family, emotional expression may have been either very restricted, or very intense. In some cases, only certain people in the house (adults) were permitted to express strong emotions in a strong fashion. The children may not have been permitted to express strong emotions, or if they did, were severely punished or abused. On the other hand, they may have participated just as fully as the adults in the emotional chaos. Children in these kinds of homes are often in an extended, never ending highly emotional, defensive, or aggressive state. Stress disordered children may be hyper reactive to other people's emotions. They just as often misinterpret or wrongly anticipate emotions in others.

The job is to help the child to experience genuine, safe, emotional freedom, but at the same time, learn the power of self control that comes from emotional regulation. This is primarily done in two ways: by our own consistent demonstration of emotional freedom and regulation when interacting with the child, and by direct, here and now instruction to the child.

Demonstrating consistent emotional freedom and regulation with a child, any child, is easier said than done. Having said that, it is important for anyone working therapeutically with children that have a stress disorder to have a clear plan for their own self care. Working with these children can be taxing not only due to their behaviors, but because of their traumatic pain as well.

It is important to be emotionally honest with children, especially those with stress disorders. Being emotionally free and honest with children does not mean "letting it all hang out" (that is what their biological family probably did). By all means, there are many adult issues and emotions that should not include children! However, it does mean that we should allow ourselves to express our genuine emotions in a controlled fashion when interacting with the child. If we are angry, show anger. If we are happy, proud, irritated, sad, show these openly. In turn, we need to give the child permission also to express their emotions. We need to help them feel safe in expressing negative emotions. We need to help them understand that negative emotions are not necessarily "bad". Show the child that while two people can be very angry with each other, they can still care for each other and they do not need to hurt each other. Focus on creating strong boundaries between your emotions, and their emotions. By doing these things, we help the child to develop a sense of their own emotions as their *own, not owned or caused by someone else*. True ownership of our own emotions is a clear sign of growing differentiation.

Direct instruction concerning emotional freedom and regulation should be an ongoing and consistent effort in treatment. One way to do this is to create a set of "emotional rights" and post them on the refrigerator, and then review them often. The list might include such things as "It is OK to be angry in this house", "You have the right to disagree", "We work issues through here" or "We compliment a job well done."

Another way of direct instruction is to educate in the "here and now." This means in the context of the emotion that is occurring. This would include citing the appropriate "emotional right" during the actual interaction, or drawing attention to how you yourself are behaving in the interaction. Praise the child when they show effort and success at emotional freedom and regulation Reminding the child frequently that you have the ability to teach and guide them in a better way of expressing their emotions, and this will help them to be successful in life is another good method.

When children learn and experience growth of healthy differentiation in a safe, supportive, environment with firm, clear limits and boundaries, they begin to heal. The child develops the a healthier ego and self identity that will allow them to become less reactive, to stand up to the stress reminders, and even perhaps, one day source of their trauma.

[QT14] Self-Harm Intervention

There are times when children begin to engage in self-harm behaviors. Sometimes, with younger children, this takes the form of head banging, hitting, slapping, or biting themselves. Older children will sometimes use sharp objects to inflict scrapes or actual cuts on their skin.

Intervention strategies for these behaviors vary, and in most cases, physical intervention such as restraint is not allowable. Also in most cases, physical restraint is not even needed. There are studies that indicate that physical restraint in self-harm cases is not productive in ending future repetitions of self-harm. Neither is raising your voice, demanding, or threatening consequences or trips to the local psychiatric hospital. So what to do?

You cannot, of course, allow a child to self-harm. Fortunately, there is an effective technique you can use to intervene in these behaviors. Listed below is an approach that will work for you. The important thing to remember is to be as consistent as possible in using the technique. It is best to use this intervention under the supervision and guidance of a behavior specialist.

The first thing you can do is to become sensitive to the child's level of stress. Most of the time, a child will begin to self-harm when they are highly stressed. In some other cases, such as with autism, the child may have a different motivation for the behavior, such as the need for stimulation, or a particular kind of stimulation. In these cases, we need to find out how to satisfy the sensory need in a more positive fashion. In the case of *stressed self-harm*, intervention should occur before these emotions get too intense, thus avoiding the behavior completely. It is a good idea to closely observe the child's behavioral signs before they begin to self-harm. If you watch closely enough, you will discover a set of signs (particular to the child) that likely present each time prior to a self-harm episode. Once a child is to the point of actually doing self-harm, the described approach will likely be less effective, so it is *very important* to *learn the child's signs of stress*.

A good intervention is to verbally recognize and name (to the child) the emotion you are seeing. Then, you can do a number of things, such as talk about the feelings, offer a different means to express the feelings (such as make a picture of the feeling), or help the child to refocus on something else, such as a preferred activity. Keeping in mind that sometimes children must accept a directive without choice, offer choice when you can. If the stress and threatened self-harm is due to a directive you gave, you might want to back off a bit, and if possible, give the child a positive choice. For example, if the child begins to self-harm after a directive to take a bath, you might first recognize their emotion ("I can see you are very angry at having to take a bath right now."), then offer a choice ("Maybe you would like to choose if you have your bath now, or after dinner.")

If the child begins to engage in self-harm, you can intervene by placing your hand, or better yet, a pillow or stuffed animal between the child's head and the wall/floor. Be sure to approach slowly, carefully, and in a non-threatening way. Get down on the floor with the child, don't stand over them. Pair this with very calm, nurturing statements to the child, such as: " I can see you are upset/angry/sad, but I sure wish you would not hurt yourself like this, I care for you and do not want to see you get hurt." *Keep repeating words to this effect!* The child may try to remove the stuffed animal, or move away from you and the toy, but be persistent in putting it back. You can do the same thing when a child is trying to scratch, slap, or hit themselves. You may want to get a special stuffed animal just for this purpose, and be sure to name it. You can also encourage the child to hug or cuddle (not hit) the stuffed animal as an alternative to their behavior. The idea here is to teach the child a more positive way to express their emotions and needs.

It is very important to pay attention to and manage your own emotions during this process. If you are expressing negative emotion or highly agitated/anxious emotion, *it will make the situation worse.* You may even find yourself thinking about physically restraining the child, *but don't do it.* In many cases, if you approach a child with the incorrect emotional expression (negative, demanding, hostile, angry), they will lash out at you when you approach. This is also true if you approach in a way that is perceived by the child to be physically threatening. If the child begins to lash out at you, simply move away. Re-examine your emotional state, expression, and behaviors. If you can tone it down, do so. If you cannot, get another adult to help who can stay calm.

Even if you are doing the technique correctly, the child may calm for a short period, and then begin their self-harm behavior again. If this happens, move in with the stuffed animal and nurturing words once again. Repeat this process until the child accepts the stuffed animal without your holding it there, and calms down. Note that you may be repeating this *many* times before the child begins to accept a new way of dealing with their emotions.

The question may be asked: What if the child is using self injury as a manipulative tool to avoid a non-preferred activity? Well, the child may do this to manipulate some of the time. In any case, you must deal with the *self-harm behavior first.* Once the child calms down, it is important to return directly back to the directive to do the non-preferred activity. Be aware that this may produce yet another round of self-harm behavior, but you must repeat the intervention *exactly* as before. It may take *many repetitions* for the child to understand that using self-harm as a manipulation will no longer work.

[QT15] The Course of Treatment for Children with PTSD

The very good news for children who suffer from Post Traumatic Stress Disorder is that their symptoms can improve to a great degree. It is important for those who care for these children to understand the course of treatment, because this understanding can help the child to progress and the caregiver to avoid frustration.

Often, adults want the symptoms of PTSD the child to be reduced quickly, not only for the child's sake, but because when a child has severe symptoms, it can be overwhelming and stressful for the caregiver. But in treating PTSD in children, the progress of the treatment cannot be rushed. When it is rushed, the child usually "shuts down", and the treatment may be delayed for some time. It is good to remember that the *child* is in charge of the pace of treatment.

Treatment makes strong use of *cognitive restructuring* and *specific adult behaviors* in working with the child. Efforts are made throughout treatment to help the child to *think differently* about themselves, their ability to deal with the world, and their relationship to their trauma. The adults who work with the child must adopt a behavioral strategy that pairs *high structure* with *high nurturing*.

The course of treatment follows roughly four stages that will overlap a great deal. The first stage of treatment is for the child to *feel completely safe in all environments*. This means "all environments": a child may feel comfortable and safe in their classroom, but not yet safe outdoors at recess, or the school rest rooms, or in the cafeteria. Helping the child to feel safe everywhere may take some length of time, depending on the nature, intensity, frequency, and duration of their trauma history. Keep in mind that we are talking at least *months*, and more likely *years*.

The second line of progress is for the child to begin to *self realize* their symptoms and level of stress. In many cases, the child has lived for so long with very high levels of stress, they do not even realize how much stress they carry. The work to help the child become self aware of their symptom processes, again, may take some time depending on the child's age, their ability to feel safe in most environments, and what their trauma was.

The midway point in treatment begins the process of *education*. The child needs to begin to learn specific techniques to help themselves to cope with the stress reaction that they now are aware of. The child needs to learn ways to access adult help in coping. This education not only includes the child, but all of the adults who work with the child, such as teachers, family, and therapeutic staff.

The last stage of treatment focuses on *stress inoculation*. This is a process of sensitively and gradually supporting the child through exposure to known stressful situations and triggers. Again, this process may take many months and even years to accomplish.

A major key to progress in treatment is that all of the adults in the child's life must gain adequate understanding of the disorder and how to approach the child. When a child encounters an adult who does not "get it", at best stress episodes increase, and at worse, treatment grinds to a halt.

[QT16] Treating Episodes of Encopresis and Enuresis in Stress Disordered Children

1. **Work at the continuing process of stress inoculation.**

   Why: The stronger the child's ego and self-esteem, the more they can manage the stress that may be one source for the wetting and soiling behaviors. When stress levels and reactivity are lessened, the wetting and soiling may become less frequent.

2. **Continue to help the child to develop healthy differentiation.**

   Why: As the child develops a clearer sense of their own identity away from the source of their trauma, they gain ego strength. The child then feels that they have a source of control inside themselves. Often, the trauma led the child to an overwhelming sense of being out of control of what was happening to them.

3. **Reassure the child when the wetting or soiling is discovered that they are not in trouble. Use a kind, firm, and neutral tone of voice.**

   Why: The child likely has had very difficult and frightening responses from adults when they wet or soil. The child may be anticipating that you too, will become very angry and perhaps punish them with some kind of abusive response.

4. **Tell the child when the wetting or soiling happens: "I don't like when you are wet or dirty. Wet and dirty belong in the toilet" Use a kind, firm, neutral tone of voice.**

   Why: The child needs to learn that the behavior is not desirable or age appropriate, but this stress inoculation must be done in a way that does not trigger a stress reaction in the child.

5. **Give the child a standard set of directives to clean up that use more or less the exact same words each time.**

   Why: The standard set of directives is to create a routine for the cleanup procedure. This also places a control on your frustration at the repeated wetting and soiling. It's only human nature to want to speak in stronger terms to "get through" to the child, but the risk is that you will begin to sound like other angry adults that may have been in their lives. Greater intensity will likely trigger a stress reaction.

6. **Make sure your directives include not only the child cleaning their body, but also taking their clothing or bed sheets to the laundry.** If they have wet or soiled carpeting, floors, or walls, be sure to have them don a pair of rubber

gloves and clean the area affected. Be sure to allow the child to bathe before they do the cleanup of the environment or the laundry. Make sure your tone of voice is kind, firm, and neutral.

Why: By having the child clean his or her body first, you demonstrate to them that they are more important than the clothing, bed, or floor. If it bothers you very much, go ahead and clean the area when they are in the tub, then have them clean the area again for "good measure".

7. **Once cleanup is complete, have a brief talk with the child:** if you sense that the wetting or soiling has its source in anger, tell the child that they are allowed to be angry, and they can learn to express their anger in a better way. If you sense that the wetting or soiling occurred due to the child having been frightened or in a stress episode, reassure the child that they have nothing to fear while in your care; you will protect them.

    Why: We need to address the (possible) cause of the behavior directly. This begins the process of the child bringing into consciousness why the behavior is happening, and that there are alternative ways to express frustration and anger, or that they have nothing to fear while in your care.

[QT 17] When a Child Begins to Share Traumatic History

Children in our care may become comfortable enough with us to begin sharing parts of their history that are traumatic. Not only can the history be painful to the child, but to us as well. It is important to know how to respond to a child who has chosen to trust us enough to tell their story.

It is hard to listen to some of the details of trauma that children may bring to us. As uncomfortable as it may be for us, it is important that we do not turn away from the child, or put them off. As the child tells us some of their history, they may enter an "emotional flood state". This means that the child may become tearful, angry, or agitated in a very intense way. Such emotional intensity may be disturbing to witness. On the other hand, the child may tell the story with what appears to be little or no emotion, leading us to wonder if the story is really true. (It likely is true).

When a child tells us their story of trauma, abuse, or neglect, the story may come out in bits and pieces that seem disjointed. Children who have experienced trauma often have inaccurate memories of the sequence of events, who was involved, and what happened to them. This also can give adults the feeling that perhaps the child is not telling the truth. (They likely are telling the truth.)

How we respond to the child when they reveal traumatic details can be very healing to the child, or it can shut the child down never to talk of it again. It is a core goal of trauma treatment to have the victim speak freely (and repeatedly) about their trauma in detail. The "therapy" of this is that each time the person tells their story, it becomes less frightening to them. Through the telling, the victim of trauma comes to a clearer understanding of their experience. Yet, is important to note that there is considerable clinical evidence that not all children benefit from telling their story repeatedly.

So, the first important thing we can do to help is to simply *listen* as the child tells their story. Our listening should be genuine; we should seek privacy for the child. We should turn off the television, and get away from other distractions. We should look at the child, and give them eye contact.

We can also encourage the child to feel comfortable and to speak by asking them simple questions during their story like: "What were you thinking when…?" or "What were you feeling when…?" You can also reflect back to them the obvious feelings that they are expressing: "You must have been very frightened and angry."

One thing many people know about traumatized children is that they may often feel like they were at fault for their own trauma. We can reassure the child at appropriate times during their story that they were not responsible for the bad things that have happened to them. We can also reassure them that their emotions, thoughts, and behaviors surrounding the traumatic event are *normal responses*; any child in their situation would have reacted the same way. The child may need specific reassurances to their trauma, such as in the case of a boy who has had a sexual trauma: "What happened to you doesn't mean you are gay." We can tell children how positive it is to talk about the trauma; how talking about it is *proven to help people*. Be sure to thank them for letting them help you.

It's OK to offer to hold the child's hand, or sit next to them, and to offer them tissues and hugs for their tears. Be sure to ask them for permission if you plan to touch them in any way. You may notice that the emotions that you see them express, while intense, (and which may include anger) are more of a genuine "release" than a threat of getting out of control.

There are several responses to the child that you *should not make*: We should not, of course, avoid or ignore the child. Do not tell the child to "wait" until they can talk to someone else. Do not allow anything to interrupt the child once they begin to tell their story. Do not give platitudes like "It's all over now, in the past, forget about it" or "You're OK now, right?" Also, be sure not to verbally *attack* the person who may have perpetrated the trauma (such as a relative). Our focus should be on the child and their emotions, not the perpetrator. Do not make promises to the child that may not be true, such as "You won't ever have to see that person again!"

While helping a child to work through their traumatic history can be uncomfortable for us, it may be one of the most compassionate, healing, and loving things we can do for the child. Be honored that the child chose *you* to tell their story to.

Appendix D: Stress Behavior Data Collection Forms

Known Stress Behaviors

Child's Name:	Date:
Time of day/duration:	Intensity: mild moderate severe (circle one)
Possible or Known Trigger:	
Behavioral Signs:	
Time of day/duration:	Intensity: mild moderate severe (circle one)
Possible or Known Trigger:	
Behavioral Signs:	
Time of day/duration:	Intensity: mild moderate severe (circle one)
Possible or Known Trigger:	
Behavioral Signs:	

Stress Behavior Observation Log

Time Before Behavior	Behavior	Time After Behavior

Child's Name _____   Date (Month/Year): _____

	1	2	3	4	5	6	7	8	9	10	11	12	13	14	15	16	17	18	19	20	21	22	23	24	25	26	27	28	29	30	31
Severe																															
Moderate																															
Mild																															
Contact																															
Number of incidents																															
duration																															

Mild, Moderate, Severe are rated according to the intensity, quality, and duration of specific stress signs presented

Contact Key

V=visit   P=phone contact   M=missed or cancelled contact
X= multiple   T=Clinician visit   C=Child Protection caseworker visit

About the Author

I grew up during the strange and turbulent 1960s and 70s in Erie, Pennsylvania. Though not 'dirt poor', my childhood family experience did not include the privileges and extravagances that I saw in the wider world. My three sisters and I were wealthy in perhaps a more important way: we had two spiritual, gentle, and firm parents in our home that was filled with love and care for each other.

My education, life experience, and vocational sense have always straddled the precarious space between secular and spiritual worlds. Having one foot planted in both worlds has allowed me to be in a unique place to meld the technical aspects of therapy with spiritual sensibilities like gentleness and compassion. My life journey has both gifted and burdened me with extensive experience in secular human services and spiritual ministry to adults, families, teens, and children.

This book was written with a passion to relieve the immense pain of children who have not had the idyllic and gentle upbringing that I had. My spirituality compels that when I see pain, I seek to heal it. If others who have similar callings read my work, perhaps more children will be healed. If others who have not yet recognized a similar calling read it, perhaps it will awaken in them at least a new awareness of the need for greater attention to these inured children.

When I begin to feel the pain of the work a bit too sharply, I try hard to be gentle with myself, and turn to my garden, or my watercolors, or to the deep woods to refresh myself. Anne, the love of my life for over thirty years, and my two fine sons, Andy and Tyler, continue to support me in my many ventures.

Each completion of a vocational task conceives and births the next... my curiosity about how to help a sexually abused child to heal their sexuality while they are still a child has grown from a passing thought in the midst of writing Gentling to my current insistent calling to apply these principles to this largely ignored area of treatment.

Bibliography

American Psychiatric Association (2000). (DSM-IV-TR) *Diagnostic and statistical manual of mental disorders, 4th edition, text revision.* Washington, DC: American Psychiatric Press, Inc.

American Psychological Association Committee on Professional Practice and Standards (1998). *Guidelines for psychological evaluations in child protection matters.*

Appellee v. Bolin, In the supreme court of Tennessee at Knoxville, No. 03S01-9508-CC-00096 (1996).

Beers, S. and DeBellis, M. (2002). Neuropsychological function in children with maltreatment related posttraumatic stress disorder. *American Journal of Psychiatry,* 159:483-486, March 2002.

Berenson, K. (2006). Childhood physical and emotional abuse by a parent: transference effects in adult personal relations. *Personality and Social Psychology Bulletin,* Vol. 32, No. 11, 1509-1522.

Berry, J., & Jobe, J. (2002). At the intersection of personality and adult development. *Journal of Research in Personality*, Vol. 36, Issue 4, 238-286.

Briere, J. & Elliott, D. (2003). Prevalence and psychological sequelae of self-reported childhood physical and sexual abuse in a general population of men and women. *Child Abuse & Neglect,* 27, 1205-1222.

Briere, J., & Elliott, D. (1997). Psychological assessment of interpersonal victimization effects in adults and children. *Psychotherapy,* Volume 34, Winter 1997, number 4.

Briere, J. (2006). Dissociative symptoms and trauma exposure: specificity, affect dysregulation and posttraumatic stress. *Journal of Nervous and Mental Disease,* Vol. 194(2), 78-82.

Briere, J., & Spinazzola, J. (2005) Phenomenology and psychological assessment of complex posttraumatic stress states. *Journal of Traumatic Stress,* Vol. 18, No. 5, 401-412.

Broderick, P. & Blewitt, P. (2006). *The Lifespan: Human Development for Helping Professionals.* Pearson Merrill Prentice Hall, New Jersey.

Bryant, R.A. (2007). Early intervention for post-traumatic stress disorder. *Early Intervention in Psychiatry,* 2007; 1: 19-26.

Carlson, B., McNutt, L., & Coi, D. (2003). Child and adult abuse among women in primary health care. *Journal of Interpersonal Violence,* Vol. 18, No. 8, 924-941.

Caspi, A. (1998). *Personality across the life course.* W. Damon (Ed.) Handbook of Child Psychology (5th Ed.). Vol. 3 Social, Emotional, and Personality Development. (pp 311-388). New York: John Wiley and Sons.

Caspi, A., & Moffitt, T.E. (1993). When do individual differences matter? A paradoxical theory of personality coherence. *Psychological Inquiry,* Vol. 4, No. 4, 247-271.

Caspi, A. & Roberts, B.W. (2001). Personality development across the life course: the argument for change and continuity. *Psychological Inquiry,* Vol. 12, No. 2, 49-66.

Ceci, S.J., & Bruck, M. (1995). *Jeopardy in the courtroom: a scientific analysis of children's testimony.* Washington, DC: American Psychological Association.

Cohen, J., Deblinger, E., Mannarino, A., & Steer, R.A. (2004). A multisite, randomized controlled trial for children with sexual abuse-related PTSD symptoms. *Journal of the American Academy of Child and Adolescent Psychiatry,* 43(4):393-402.

Cox, B., MacPherson, P., Enns, M., and McWilliams, L. (2004). Neuroticism and self-criticism associated with posttraumatic stress disorder in a nationally representative sample. *Behavior Research and Therapy.* Vol. 42, Issue 1, 105-114.

Crouch, J.L., Smith, D.W., & Ezzell, C.E. (1999). Measuring reactions to sexual trauma among children: comparing the children's impact of traumatic events scale and the trauma symptom checklist for children. *Child Maltreatment,* 1999.

Daud, A., Klinteberg, B., and Rydelius, P. (2008). Trauma, PTSD and personality: the relationship between prolonged traumatization and personality impairments. *Scandinavian Journal of Caring Sciences.*

DeBellis, M. (1999). Developmental Traumatology: Neurological Development in Maltreated Children with PTSD. *Child Maltreatment,* September 1999, Vol. XVI, Issue 9.

Depue, R.., & Collins, P. (1999). Neurobiology of the structure of personality: dopamine, facilitation of incentive motivation, and extraversion. *Behavioral and Brain Sciences,* 22;491-569.

Depue, R. (1995). Neurobiological factors in personality and depression. *European Journal of Personality*, Vol. 9, Issue 5, 413-439.

Englehard, I., van den Hout, M., & Kindt, M. (2003). The relationship between neuroticism, pre-traumatic stress, and post-traumatic stress: a prospective study. *Personality and Individual Differences*. Vol. 35, Issue 2, 381-388.

Erickson, S. (1999). Somatization as an indicator of trauma adaptation in long-term pediatric cancer survivors. *Clinical Child Psychology and Psychiatry*, Vol. 4, No. 3, 415-426.

Fauerbach, J., Lawrence, J., Schmidt, C., Munster, A, and Costa, P. (2000) Personality predictors of injury related posttraumatic stress disorder. *Journal of Nervous &Mental Disease*. 188(8):510-517.

Finding words: half a nation by 2010 interviewing children and preparing for court. (June 2003). Retrieved June 1, 2007 from http://www.ndaa.org/pdf/finding_words_2003.pdf.

Fonagy, P. (1999). Male Perpetrators of Violence Against Women: An Attachment Theory Perspective. *Journal of Applied Psychoanalytic Studies*, Vol. 1, No. 1.

Ford, J., Racusin, R., Ellis, C., Daviss, W., Reiser, J., Fleischer, A., & Thomas, J. (2000). Child maltreatment, other trauma exposure, and posttraumatic symptomology among children with oppositional defiant disorder and attention deficit hyperactivity disorder. *Child Maltreatment*, Vol. 5, No. 3, 2005-217.

Foster, J., & MacQueen, G. 2008. Neurobiological factors linking personality traits and major depression. *Canadian Journal of Psychiatry*, 53(1):6-13.

Heim, C., Newport, J., Bonsall, R., Miller, A., & Meneroff, C. (2001). Altered pituitary-adrenal axis responses to provocative challenge tests in adult survivor of child abuse. *American Journal of Psychiatry,* 158:575-581.

Heinrivh, M., Wagner, D., Schoch, W., Soravia, L., Hellhammer, D., and Ehlert, U. (2005). Predicting posttraumatic stress symptoms from pretraumatic stress risk factors: a 2- year prospective follow-up study in firefighters. *American Journal of Psychiatry*, 162:2276-2286.

Hishaw-Fuselier, S., Heller, S., Parton, V., Robinson, L., & Boris, N. (2004). Trauma and Attachment: the case for Disrupted Attachment Disorder. J.D. Osofsky (Ed.), *Young children and trauma: intervention and treatment.* (pp. 47-68). New York: The Guilford Press.

Hunt, N., & Gakenyi, M. (2005). Comparing refugee and nonrefugees: the Bosnian experience. *Journal of Anxiety Disorders*. Vol. 19, Issue 6, 717-723.

Jumper, S.A. (1995). A meta-analysis of the relationship of child sexual abuse to adult psychological adjustment. *Child Abuse & Neglect*, 19, 715-728.

Kagan, J. (2000). Temperament. In A. Kazdin (Ed.), *Encyclopedia of Psychology*. New York: Oxford University Press.

Kamalla, L., Bruck, M., Ceci, S.J., & Shuman, D.W. (2005). Disclosure of child sexual abuse: what does research tell us about the ways that children tell? *Psychology, Public Policy, and Law,* 2005, Vol. 11, No. 1, 194-226.

Kaplow, J.B., Dodge, K.A., Amaya-Jackson, L., & Saxe, G.N. (2005). Pathways to PTSD, part II: sexually abused children. *American Journal of Psychiatry,* 162:1305-1310.

Knezevic, G., Opacic, G., Savic, D., and Priebe, S. (2005). Do personality traits predict post-traumatic stress: A prospective study in civilians experiencing air attacks. *Psychological Medicine*, 35:659-663.

Koenen, K. C. (2006) Self-regulation as a central mechanism. Psychobiology of Posttraumtic Stress Disorder: A Decade of Progress. Vol. 1071: 255-266.

Lauterbach, D. (2001). Personality profiles of trauma survivors. *Traumatology*, Vol. 7, No. 1.

Lauterbach, D., & Vrana, S. (2001). The relationship among personality variables, exposure to traumatic events, and severity of posttraumatic stress symptoms. *Journal of Traumatic Stress*, Vol. 14, No. 1, 29-45.

Lecic-Tosevski, D., Gavrilovic, J., Knezevic, G., and Priebe, S. 2003. Personality factors and posttraumatic stress: associations in civilians one year after air attacks. *Journal of Personality Disorders,* Vol. 17, Issue 6, 537-549.

Lester, P., Wong, S., Hendren, R. (2003). The Neurobiological Effects of Trauma. *Adolescent Psychiatry.*

Lieberman, A.F., & Van Horn, P. (2004) Assessment and treatment of young children exposed to traumatic events. J.D. Osofsky (Ed.), *Young children and trauma: intervention and treatment.* (pp.111-138). New York: The Guilford Press.

Lombardo, T.W., & Gray, M.J. (2005). Beyond exposure for posttraumatic stress disorder (PTSD symptoms. *Behavior Modification,* Vol. 29, No. 1, 3-9.

Marshal, R.D., Spitzer, R., & Liebowitz, M.R. (1999). Review and critique of the new DSM-IV diagnosis of acute stress disorder. *Journal of Psychiatry,* 156:1677-1685.

May, J. (2005). Family attachment narrative therapy: healing the experience of early childhood maltreatment. *Journal of Marital and Family Therapy,* July 2005.

McAdams, D., Bauer, J., Sakaeda, A., Anyidoho, N, Machado, M., Magrino-Failla, K., White, K., and Pals, J. (2006). Continuity and change in the life story: a longitudinal study of autobiographical memories in emerging adulthood. *Journal of Personality*, Vol. 74, Issue 5, 1371-1400.

Mrockek, D.K., & Spiro, A. (2003). The Journals of Gerontology Series B: Psychological Sciences and Social Sciences, 58:P153-P165.

Muller, R., Sicoli, L., & Lemieux, K. (2000). Relationship between attachment style and post traumatic stress symptomology among adults who report the experience of childhood abuse. *Journal of Traumatic Stress*, Vo. 13, No. 2.

Nader, K. (2001) Treatment Methods for Childhood Trauma. In Wilson, J.P., Friedman, M.J., & Lindy, J.D. (Eds.) *Treating psychological trauma & PTSD* (pp.278-334). New York: The Guilford Press.

Neuman, D.A., Houskamp, B.M., Pollock, V.E., & Briere, J. (1996). The long term sequelae of childhood sexual abuse in women: a meta-analytic review. *Child Maltreatment*, 1,6-16.

Paris, J. (2005). Neurobiological dimensional models of personality: a review of the models of Cloninger, Depue, and Siever. *Journal of Personality Disorders*, Volume 19, Issue 2, 156-170.

People v. Stritzinger, 34 Cal. 3d 505, 668 P.2d 738, 194 Cal. Rptr. 431 (1983).

Perry, B., & Azad, I. (1999). Post-traumatic Stress Disorders in children and adolescents. *Current opinions in Pediatrics,* Volume 11, number 4: (August 1999).

Perry, B. (2001b). The neurodevelopmental impact of violence in childhood. In Schetky D & Benedek, E. (Eds.) *Textbook of child and adolescent forensic psychiatry.* Washington, D.C.: American Psychiatric Press, Inc. (221-238)

Perry, B. Neurobiological sequelae of childhood of childhood trauma: post traumatic stress disorders in children. In: *Catecholamine Function in Post Traumatic Stress Disorder: Emerging Concepts* (M. Murburg, Ed.) American Psychiatric Press, Washington, D.C., 253-276, 1994.

Perry, B., & Pollard, D. Altered brain development following global neglect in early childhood. *Society For Neuroscience: Proceedings from Annual Meeting*, New Orleans, 1997.

Perry, B.. Neurobiological sequelae of childhood trauma: post traumatic stress disorders in children. In: *Catecholamine Function in Post Traumatic Stress Disorder: Emerging Concepts* (M. Murburg, Ed.) American Psychiatric Press, Washington, DC, 253-276, 1994.

Perry, B. (1996). *Violence and childhood trauma: Understanding and responding to the effects of violence on young children.* Grund Foundation Publishers, Cleveland, Ohio. 1996, pp. 67-80.

Perry, B.. & Pollard, D. Altered brain development following global neglect in early childhood. *Society For Neuroscience: Proceedings from Annual Meeting,* New Orleans, 1997.

Psychological first aid: filed operations guide, 2nd edition. (July 2006). Retrieved June 1, 2007 from http://www.ncptsd.va.gov/ncmain/ncdocs/manuals/smallerPFA_2ndEditionwi thappendices.pdf.

Regan, J. Johnson, C., & Alderson, A. (2002) *Expert testimony linking child sexual abuse with posttraumatic stress disorder.* April 2002.

Richeters, M.M. and Volkmar, F.R. (1994). Reactive Attachment Disorder of Early Childhood. *J. Am. Acad. Child Adolesc. Psychiatry,* 33, 3: 328-332.

Roberts, B.W., Mroczek, D. (2008). Personality trait change in adulthood. *Current Directions in Psychological Science,* Vol. 17, No. 1, 31-35(5).

Roberts, B.W., DelVecchio, W.F. (2000). The rank-order consistency of personality traits from childhood to old age: a quantitative review of longitudinal studies. *Psychological Bulletin,* Vol. 126, No. 1, 3-25.

Roberts, B.W., Wood, D., Smith, J.L. (2005). Evaluating five factor theory and social investment perspectives on personality trait development. *Journal of Research in Personality,* 39, 166-184.

Ruchkin, V., Schwab-Stone, M., Koposov, R. Vermeiren, R., and Steiner, H. (2002). Violence exposure, posttraumatic stress, and personality in juvenile delinquents. *Journal of the American Academy of Child & Adolescent Psychiatry.* 41(3):322-329.

Schuder, M.R., & Lyons-Ruth, K. (2004). "Hidden trauma" in infancy: Attachment, fearful arousal, and early dysfunction of the stress response system. In J.D. Osofsky (Ed.), *Young children and trauma: intervention and treatment.* (pp. 69-106). New York: The Guilford Press.

Schore, A. (2002). Dysregulation of the right brain: a fundamental mechanism of traumatic attachment and the psychopathogenesis of posttraumatic stress disorder. *Australian and New Zealand Journal of Psychiatry,* 36(1):9-30, February 2002.

Schore, Allan, (2001) The effects of early relational trauma on right brain development, affect regulation, & infant mental health. *Infant Mental Health Journal,* 22, 201-269.

Schuder, M, and Lyons-Ruth, K. (2001). Hidden Trauma in Infancy. In Wilson, J.P., Friedman, M.J., & Lindy, J.D. (Eds.) *Treating psychological trauma & PTSD* (pp.69-104). New York: The Guilford Press.

Schwedtfeger, K.L. & Goff, B.S.N. (2007). Intergenerational transmission of trauma: exploring mother-infant prenatal attachment. *Journal of Traumatic Stress*, 20, 39-51.

Starasburger, L.H., Gutheil, T.J., & Brodsky, A. (1997). On wearing two hats: role conflict in serving as both psychotherapist and expert witness. *American Journal of Psychiatry*, 154:4, April 1997.

Vander Kolk, B. (1998) Re-enactment, Revictimization, and Masochism. *Psychiatric Clinics of North America*, Vol. 12, No. 2, 389-411. June, 1998.

Van Voorhees, Elizabeth. (2004). The effects of child maltreatment on the hypothalamic-pituitary-adrenal axis. *Trauma, Violence, & Abuse*, Vol. 5, No. 4, 333-352.

Victims of Child Abuse Act of 1990, Article IV.

Walters, J.T.R., Bisson, J.I., & Shepherd, J.P. (2006). Predicting post-traumatic stress disorder: validation of the trauma screening questionnaire in victims of assault. *Psychological Medicine*, 37, 143-150.

Warner, Megan B., Morey, Leslie C., Finch, John F., Gunderson, John G., Skodol, Andrew, Sanislow, Charles A., Shea, Tracie M., McGlashan, Thomas H., and Grilo, Carlos M. (2004). The longitudinal relationship of personality traits and disorders. *Journal of Abnormal Psychology*, 113:217-227.

Watters, T., Brineman, J., Wright, S. (2007). Between a rock and a hard place: why hearsay testimony may be a necessary evil in child sexual abuse cases. *Journal of Forensic Psychology Practice,*. Volume: 7, Issue: 1.

Weine, S.M., Becker, D.F., Vojvoda, D., Hodzic, E., Sawyer, M., Hyman, L., Laub, D., and McGlashan, T.H. (2005) Individual change after genocide in Bosnian survivors of "ethnic cleansing": assessing personality dysfunction. *Journal of Traumatic Stress*, Vol. 11, No. 1, 147-153.

Wilson, J.P. (2001) An overview of clinical considerations and principles in the treatment of PTSD. In Wilson, J.P., Friedman, M.J., & Lindy, J.D. (Eds.) *Treating psychological trauma & PTSD* (pp.59-93). New York: The Guilford Press.

Wexler, R., (1995). *Wounded innocents*. Buffalo: Prometheus Books.

Wrightsman, L.S. (2005). *Forensic Psychology*. USA: Wadsworth.

Wonderlich, S.A., Crosby, R.D., Mitchell, J.E., Thompson, K., Smyth, J.M., Redlin, J., and Jones-Paxton, M. (2001). Sexual trauma and personality:

developmental vulnerability and additive effects. *Journal of Personality Disorders*, Vol. 15, Issue 15, 496-504.

Young, S.N., Moskowitz, D.S. (2005). Serotonin and affiliative behavior. *Behavioral and Brain Sciences*, 28:367-368.

Zald, D.H., & Depue, R.A. Serotonergic functioning correlates with positive and negative affect in psychiatrically healthy males. *Personality and Individual Differences*, Vol. 30, Issue 1, 71-86.

Index

A

accepting nurturing, 97
acting out, 194
Acute Stress, 6, 14, 15, 30, 43, 45, 46, 151, 152, 154, 178, 183, 197
ADHD, 20, 30, 43, 183
affect dysregulation, 174
affection, 92
age normal development, 65, 66
allostatic behavioral signs, 31–32
allostatic load, 15–16
anal penetration, 27, 171
anger, 28, 113, 119, 179, 186
Attention-Deficit Hyperactivity Disorder. *See* ADHD
avoidance, 3, 11, 16, 174

B

baby talk, 26, 33, 38, 185
bedwetting alarm, 170
behavior modification, 79–82
bi-polar disorder, 12, 20, 30, 43, 99
borderline personality disorder, 12, 99
Bowen, B., 47

C

Child Sexual Abuse Accommodation Syndrome, 73, 133, 141, 180
Child Stress Profile. *See* CSP
classroom protocols, 151–53
cognitive-behavioral techniques, 65
compassion fatigue, 157
compliments, 93–94
confabulation, 176–77
countertransference, 157

CSP, 10–12
    and children under 5, 12
    case study, 12–14
cues. *See* triggers
cutting, 93, 120

D

Da Costa, J.M., 5
data collection, 145–50
DDAVP, 27, 28, 169
decompensation, 27, 47, 74, 75
desensitization, 159, 160
desire to please, 176
detachment, 3, 11, 16, 174
developmental regressions, 20, 63
differentiation, 47, 48, 58, 59, 67, 96, 179, 205
    healthy, 197–200
dignity, 105–6
dissociative state, 21, 53

E

ego structure, 34, 185
ego structure damage, 175
ego wrapping, 4, 8, 38, 47, 61
emotional attending, 94–95
emotional release, 38
empathy, 13, 24, 33, 40, 65, 71, 72, 91, 95, 106, 107, 108, 109, 165, 184, 186
encopresis, 19, 28, 113–14, 171–72, 178–79, 186, 205–6
enuresis, 28, 113–14, 169–70, 178–79, 186, 205–6
escalation, 37
exhaustion/return, 38
externalizers, 49
eye contact, 95–96

F

familly preservation, 141–44
feces
    animal, 31, 183
    defense mechanism, 178
    manipulation. *See* feces smearing
    sensation, 171
feces smearing, 19, 27, 113, 165, 171, 178
flashback. *See* re-experiencing
flat affect, 21, 22, 24, 37, 39
flight behavior, 37
foster care, viii, 6–8, 9, 12–14, 26, 39, 65, 174, 180–
    82

G

Galvanic Skin Resistance monitor. *See* GSR
gentling
    defined, 1–2
    technique vs. quality, 67
grief, 6, 48, 49, 68, 143
GSR, 14

H

hallucination, 28, 165
head banging, 120, 121, 166, 201
hiding behaviors, 21, 37, 59, 60, 187
humor, 93
hyperactive, 187
hyperactivity, 31, 183, 217
hypersensitive, 13
hypervigilance, 25, 33, 45, 59, 187

I

IEP, 152
Individualized Education Plan. *See* IEP
internalizers, 49

J

journal, 160

L

light switch effect, 20

M

masturbation, 84, 166, 180, 184
mental retardation, 27

N

negative engagement, 99–101
nightmares, 13, 16, 31, 32, 80, 113, 165, 183, 184,
    186
nighttime diapers, 169, 171
numbing, 3, 11, 16, 186

O

oppositional defiant disorder, 30, 154, 180

P

panic attack, 3
phantom pain, 176
physical boundary problems, 34, 185
physiological signs, 20–21
play engagement, 110
positive re-engagement, 66–69
precocious, 70, 188
psychobiological alterations, 11
psycho-education, 42
PTSD, 174–75
    and confabulation, 176–77
    and foster care, 73, 180–82
    defined, 6
    secondary, 6
    treatment plan, 9
    trust and intimacy, 16
pupil dilation, 21, 37, 187

Q

Quick Teach sheets, viii, *See* Appendix C

R

RAD, 24, 46, 180
rage, 28
rape
    witness, 76
Reactive Attachment Disorder. *See* RAD
reconnection, 69–72

re-experiencing, 11, 16, 32, 174, 184
relational problems, 34, 185
respect, 105–6, 191
risk taking, 119, 120, 187
Rogers, F., ix, 103, 109

S

Schnarch, D., 47, 58
secondary traumatization, 157
secrecy, 133–37
Sedwick, H., ix
self-harm, 119–24, 188
    anger, 121
    as manipulation, 123
    interventions, 201–2
self-realizing, 42
sexual self-stimulation, 21, 124
sexual trauma, 83–85
sexualized behaviors, 187
sexually precocious, 21, 22, 181
sexually precocious knowledge, 32, 184
sleep disorders, 31
sleep disturbance, 16
sleep medication, 170, 172
soiling, 19, 27, 28, 32, 37, 38, 113, 114, 165, 171,
    172, 178, 198, 205, 206
stress break, 52, 154, 155, 193–95
stress episode, 120
    eye contact, 96
    vs. tantrum, 35, 117
stress inoculation, 42
    healthy differentiation, 197–200
stress load, 15, 38, 58, 93
stress reactivity, 7, 14, 17, 40, 41, 52, 58, 60, 61, 107,
    122, 139–40, 142, 143, 147, 149, 159
stress tolerance, 21, 80
structure
    importance of, 91

Summit, R., 133
suppository, 171

T

tantrums, 117
target fascination, 75, 128
tattling, 196
team approaches, 115
tickling, 34, 185
transference, 26, 119, 130, 157, 158, 165, 176, 215
trauma, 3–8
    defined, 3
    sexual, 83–85
traumatic memory, 127–32
treatment plan, 9, 42, 44, 57, 88, 159, 194
triggers, 13–16, 31, 39, 46–48, 107, 193
    people as, 139–40

U

unconditional positive regard, 96–97
unindulgent favor, 94
urine
    absorbtion, 169
    cleanup, 81
    defense mechanism, 178

V

vocal changes, 21
voice tones, 52, 61, 85, 103

W

wet wipes, 28
wetting, 13, 14, 19, 27, 28, 32, 33, 37, 38, 81, 82,
    113, 114, 165, 169, 178, 185, 205, 206

What if we could resolve childhood trauma early, rather than late?

We are understanding more and more about how early traumatic experiences affect long-term mental and physical health:

• Physical impacts are stored in muscles and posture
• Threats of harm are stored as tension
• Overwhelming emotion is held inside
• Negative emotional patterns become habit
• Coping and defense mechanism become inflexible

What if we could resolve childhood trauma before years go by and these effects solidify in body and mind?

In a perfect world, we'd like to be able to shield children from hurt and harm. In the real world, children, even relatively fortunate ones, may experience accidents, injury, illness, and loss of loved ones. Children unfortunate enough to live in unsafe environments live through abuse, neglect, and threats to their well-being and even their life.

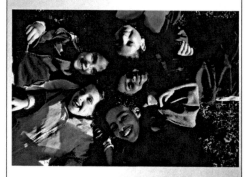

Children and
Traumatic Incident Reduction:
Creative and Cognitive Approaches

Edited by Marian K. Volkman, CTS, CMF

Experts Praise *Children and TIR*

"This book is a must for any therapist working with kids. Naturally, it focuses on the approach of Traumatic Incident Reduction, but there is a lot of excellent material that will be useful even to the therapist who has never before heard of TIR and may not be particularly interested in learning about it. The general approach is respectful of clients, based on a great deal of personal experience by contributors as well as on the now extensive research base supporting TIR, and fits the more general research evidence on what works".

—Robert Rich, PhD

"Much useful and thoroughly researched information is packed into this priceless volume in the TIR Application Series. This is a good book for parents to read because s/he may take away an understanding of the many different therapy strategies available to them and their children."

—Lisa Bullert, *Reader Views*

ISBN 978-1-932690-30-9　　　　**List $19.95**
More information at www.TIRbook.com

REPAIR For Kids

Recognition
Entry
Process
Awareness
Insight
Rhythm

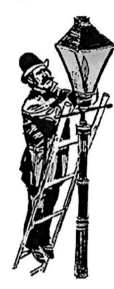

Enter a **Six-Stage Program** with your child to cross the Bridge of Recovery and make available a whole new world of hope:

• Uncover and acknowledge feelings by discovering emotion
• Build self-esteem and optimism with the "Magic Mirror"
• Discern healthy and unhealthy messages
• Learn self-soothing skills with "Dear Diary" letters to the inner-child
• Reveal inner states with picture drawing
• Break free from the confines of false shame
• Cultivate self-care skills and practices
• Learn about boundaries and bodies
• Return to the natural rhythm and flow of life

"*REPAIR for Kids* provides a comprehensive, honest and passionate approach for children recovering from sexual abuse. Children will benefit from this book, and be encouraged to continue on their recovery journey."
—Jill Osborne, Ed.S,
author of *Sam Feels Better Now*

"I wish I had had something like this a long time ago for my sad and shamed 'little girl' within. I can't think of anything I'd change. You have covered it all and with wonderful sensitivity, perfect timing and terrific repair exercises. I love the cartoons and the colorfulness of your book as well."
—Marcelle Taylor, MFT

ISBN 978-1-932690-57-6   List $34.95
More information at www.TheLamplighters.org

Breinigsville, PA USA
29 August 2009
223187BV00004B/1/P